KISS SLEEPING BEAUTY GOOD-BYE

Kiss Sleeping Beauty Good-Bye

Breaking the Spell of Feminine Myths and Models

Madonna Kolbenschlag

Doubleday & Company, Inc.
Garden City, New York

Library of Congress Cataloging in Publication Data

Kolbenschlag, Madonna, 1935–
Kiss sleeping beauty good-bye.

Includes bibliographical references and index.
1. Women—Psychology. 2. Sex role in literature.
3. Self-actualization (Psychology). 4. Self-realization. 5. Feminism. I. Title.
HQ1206.K59 301.41'2
ISBN: 0-385-14186-6
Library of Congress Catalog Card Number 78–68346

Grateful acknowledgment is made to the following publishers for permission to quote from their published works:

Doubleday & Company, Inc. for *The Three Marias: New Portuguese Letters,* by Maria Isabel Barreno, Maria Teresa Horta, Maria Velho da Costa, trans. Helen Lane, Copyright © 1975 by Doubleday & Company, Inc.

From *Conversations: Working Women Talk About Doing a "Man's Job,"* edited by Terry Wetherby, Copyright © 1977 by Terry Wetherby. Reprinted with permission of Les Femmes Publishing, Millbrae, California.

Quotations from "Prayer for Revolutionary Love" and "Divorcing" from Denise Levertov, *The Freeing of the Dust,* Copyright © 1975 by Denise Levertov. Reprinted by permission of New Directions.

From *Surfacing* by Margaret Atwood, Copyright © 1972 by Margaret Atwood. Reprinted by permission of Simon and Schuster, Inc., a Division of Gulf & Western Corporation.

Quotations from *Becoming Woman* by Penelope Washbourn, Copyright © 1977 by Penelope Washbourn. Reprinted with permission of Harper & Row, Publishers, Inc.

Quotations from *The Uses of Enchantment: The Meaning and Importance of Fairy Tales,* by Bruno Bettelheim, Copyright © 1976 by Bruno Bettelheim. Reprinted by permission of Alfred A. Knopf, Inc. Portions of this book originally appeared in *The New Yorker.*

For Maud Cecilia Mathews Kolbenschlag,
and all my sisters—everywhere.

ACKNOWLEDGMENTS

To properly acknowledge all whose influence has impressed these pages would be a hopeless task. A book like *Kiss Sleeping Beauty Good-Bye* is never a monologue; it is a record of a long conversation with countless others whose impact on my own thought I have perhaps even forgotten. But every book owes its existence to providential persons whose faith in the author transforms an idea into a reality. For this, I am especially grateful to Judy Ress, John A. Miles, Jr., and Deborah McCann. Nor would any of the words herein ever have seen print without the editorial guidance of John Breslin, S.J., and the help of that unsung secretarial sisterhood, without whom the work of the world—as we know it—would grind to a halt. Thank you, Kathy Kiritsis, Bobbi Thompson, Janet Wright and Carmela Rulli.

CONTENTS

INTRODUCTION

The ancients debated the question of whether or not woman could have a soul. Today the "woman question" is one of removing the barriers that prevent woman from *becoming* a soul. This book concerns itself with the obstacles to self-actualization, transcendence and redemption that constitute the challenge of being female—and at the same time, of being fully human—in the contemporary era. If it has any uniqueness in the chorus of voices that have already spoken on the subject, it is that this work assumes the perspective of faith. It is addressed to those who are believers in the transcendent purpose of life, who identify themselves with the great religious traditions. It is also addressed to those who are not believers, offering them a challenging vision that confirms the emerging autonomy of women as the fulfillment of a destiny that transcends the personal and the temporal.

From the vantage point of the twenty-first century, we will no doubt regard the "women's movement" as possibly the most significant and consequential social phenomenon of the present era. Within that movement, the articulation of the spirituality of women has understandably come late. For how can we know our destiny until we see what we are capable of? Much testing, much reflecting, much living must intervene before we can say, "My soul is now my own." This is finally what *liberation* means, that I have rescued my spirit from repressive coercion, from inner compulsion and from the hazards of freedom itself.

My book is the fruit of many conversations with women, of many years spent in teaching them, of many months of research, of many more hours spent in contemplating what it means to be a woman. It is not meant to be a book of abstract concepts or prescriptions, but a record of experience—a map of collective as well as personal discovery and discernment. Its primary authority is that it is being lived by women today.

Much of what we live by and attribute to nature or destiny is, in reality, a pervasive cultural mythology. Because myths are no less powerful than nature and because they mirror as well as model our existence, I have introduced six familiar fairy tales as heuristic devices for interpreting the experience of women. These tales are parables of what women have become; and at the same time, prophecies of the spiritual metamorphosis to which they are called.

No doubt these words will appeal primarily to those accustomed to finding insight, solace and challenge in books. Yet millions of women and men who have neither the resources, nor the leisure, nor the possibilities of those who are likely to read this book are also the object of its message. The first step toward liberating them must be to liberate ourselves, for we are all culture-bound prisoners of our own time.

The faith that is expressed here, and that is asked of women and men who would be truly free, is not backward-looking or nostalgic; nor is it blindly iconoclastic and memoryless. It nurtures the seed of our future becoming in the revelation of the present, in a tradition that remains faithful to itself by transcending itself.

September 12, 1978

KISS SLEEPING BEAUTY GOOD-BYE

the legend

Woman is the Sleeping Beauty, Cinderella, Snow White, she who receives and submits. In song and story the young man is seen departing adventurously in search of a woman; he slays the dragon, he battles giants; she is locked in a tower, a palace, a garden, a cave, she is chained to a rock, a captive, sound asleep: she waits.

—Simone de Beauvoir, *The Second Sex*[1]

Whether it is Snow White in her glass coffin or Sleeping Beauty on her bed, the adolescent dream of everlasting youth and perfection is just that: a dream. The alteration of the original curse, which threatened death, to one of prolonged sleep suggests that the two are not all that different. If we do not want to change and develop, then we might as well remain in a deathlike sleep. During their sleep the heroines' beauty is a frigid one; theirs is the isolation of narcissism. In such self-involvement which excludes the rest of the world there is no suffering, but also no knowledge to be gained, no feelings to be experienced.

—Bruno Bettelheim, *The Uses of Enchantment*[2]

"I feel as if I've been sleepwalking through my life. As if I'm Sleeping Beauty and still haven't wakened up."

—Clarissa, in Marilyn French's *Women's Room*[3]

Each of us has a favorite bedtime story or two from childhood, one that our parents or nannies had to repeat over and over to satisfy our greedy imaginations, one that we never tired of and came to identify with ourselves, one that probably lies faded and dog-eared in the attic of our memory. Sometimes it is a fairy tale or a Mother Goose story, a Golden Book or a children's novel. Sometimes it is a story made up by a desperate parent; sometimes it is a story we have made up. Recalled in later years, it can be a kind of prism of the self: reflecting what we think of ourselves as well as what we have made of ourselves. Like Charles Foster Kane's *Rosebud,* it can reveal the "missing piece" of our personality. Whether it is *The Ugly Duckling* or *The Little Engine That Could,* its persistence in our memory speaks volumes about who and what we are, and what we are becoming.

Fairy tales are the bedtime stories of the collective consciousness. They persist in the cultural memory because they interpret crises of the human condition that are common to all of us. They are shared wish fulfillments, abstract dreams that resolve conflicts and give meaning to experience. Philosophers of myth have sketched the genealogy of fairy tales, tracing most of them back to primitive *rites de passage* and initiation rituals. In some way, most of them celebrate the metaphoric death of the old inadequate self as it is about to be reborn on a higher plane of existence. Like Charon's boat, they grant us passage to a world where the mortal and the eternal, the sacred and the secular, meet; where the past and the future are divined; where good and evil clash, but where goodness, truth and beauty are destined to victory. Fairy tales are thus primarily metaphors of the human personality, of the individual psyche's struggle to be free of fear and compulsion.

The omnipresence of myths and fairy tales in so many aspects of culture—speech idioms, poetry, music, dance, painting, sculpture, drama, fiction, film—suggests that these stories describe and narrate the structures of a collective as well as individual experience. The fairy tale, especially, may be emblematic of predisposing conditions of a particular social milieu. The fact that most fairy tales embody elements associated with the archetypal "feminine" points to the possibility that they recapitulate a view of reality that is rooted in the determinism of sex roles.

It is significant that approximately one third of the original Grimm collection came from a single old nurse, "alte Maria," and that the Grimms were the first to attempt to retell the fairy tales as they had first been told by mothers and female caretakers of children. The Grimms were contemporaries of Bachofen (there is some evidence that they had the same teachers) who popularized a theory of a female-centered prehistory of classical civilization. Thus, the fairy tales are unique parables of feminine socialization and graphic examples of a cultural consciousness that predates the emergence of women into their full stature as persons.

One of the most familiar, most often repeated, most often metamorphosed fairy tales in Western culture is the story of Sleeping Beauty. Singular because of its multiple variants, the tale nevertheless contains certain elements that are common to most versions:

1. The birth of a beautiful female infant after years of generative sterility.
2. A forgotten goddess, a slighted god or fairy godmother, a jealous queen—a principle of EVIL.
3. A revenge curse.
4. A lethal spindle and a pricked finger at puberty.
5. A sleep of a hundred years—the result of the good fairy godmother's intervention, moderating the curse of death, a principle of GOOD.
6. An impassable hedge of thorns.
7. The collective sleep of the kingdom: the fate of a people is bound up with the fate of the heroine.
8. Unmarried king or prince, destined to save Sleeping Beauty and her people—the expected OTHER.
9. The kiss that awakens Sleeping Beauty.

At the psychological level, the tale is a recognizable parable of the onset of puberty and the confrontation with sexuality. It sets "limits" and introduces the superego as a check to libido. The "Briar Rose" variants in particular emphasize the "hedge of thorns," the protective wall that surrounds the passive heroine. Bettelheim's interpretation illuminates the subjective-developmental aspect of the story: He sees the "sleep" as a kind of narcissistic withdrawal in the face of the stresses of adolescence (symbolized by the shedding of blood after touching the distaff). The story serves as a warning that failure to relate positively to "the other" may lead to a comatose existence in which the entire world becomes dead to the person.

An examination of the variants of the tale reveals some interesting contrasts in emphasis. In general, the Perrault and Grimm versions portray the "sleep" as a concentration of powers, a period of quiet preparation for fulfillment and an exclusive relation to an ultimate Other. In these versions, *being* is idealized.

A significant variation of the Sleeping Beauty motif occurs in Wagner's *Ring of the Nibelung* based on the Germanic saga, the *Nibelungenlied*. Brünhilde, the warrior-maiden, is punished for attempting to aid the hero, Siegmund. Wotan—the patriarch of the gods—casts a spell of "sleep" over his daughter, and surrounds her with a wall of fire until the destined hero penetrates it and awakens her with a kiss. In *Die Walküre,* as she succumbs to the "sleep," Wotan sings the refrain, "Thus the god takes away your godhead." Significantly, when Siegfried (the destined hero) approaches the sleeping Brünhilde, he removes her magic armor—she awakes to his kiss as a mortal woman, no longer a "god," her strength and power diminished. Thus, the opera version seems to emphasize the patriarchal repression of assertive autonomy and the assumption of power by a female. In contrast to the other versions where beauty—*being*—is idealized, and revenge is based on envy, in this cycle of tales, *doing* (usurping a male prerogative) is punished and romantic vulnerability (femininity) is celebrated.

Thus, at the universal level of meaning, Sleeping Beauty is most of all a symbol of *passivity,* and by extension a metaphor for the spiritual condition of women—cut off from autonomy and transcendence, from self-actualization and ethical capacity in a male-dominated milieu. But this is to restrict the meaning of the metaphoric image to its descriptive content. Its very persistence in the cultural context suggests that the story has a phoenixlike aspect. Out of the ashes of cultural memory, out of the recognition of the metaphor as descriptive of a universal condition that is passing, arises a dynamic symbol calling women forth to an "awakening" and to spiritual maturity.

And, as in the fairy tale, the Kingdom of God waits.

ONE

Sleeping Beauty at Seventeen

YOU see them in high school study halls, twisting their tresses and staring out the window. You see them in offices, filing stacks of reports and glancing at the clock anxiously. You see them in laundromats, in supermarkets, in beauty parlors, on buses. You see them on the couch, TV blaring, paging through *Seventeen* magazine. Wherever you see them, they are young, anxious, languid, bored, unsatisfied with themselves. (And when they are no longer young their boredom has changed to self-hatred and their anxiety to depression.) They all have one thing in common: They are convinced they are waiting for something. They imagine themselves in a state of readiness, of expectancy, of waiting for life and for their real existence to begin. In fact, it has already begun—it is passing them by, while their energies atrophy. They are sleeping beauties who may never wake up.

> For the upbringing we have had is that of overbred female setters, female pointers—specially trained to freeze in our tracks when we flush game.
>
> —*The Three Marias: New Portuguese Letters,*
> Maria Isabel Barreno, Maria Teresa Horta,
> Maria Velho da Costa

Where does it all begin? It begins with the fantasies of a young man or woman about their unborn child. Parental projections begin to affect the unborn female long before she becomes a reality in the lives of her parents. Unborn children, particularly the first-born, are usually sexualized in our fantasies in the dominant, or male gender. Pregnancy guides and doctors talk about "him." (Books on infant care will concede an occasional "her.") More importantly, Mom and Dad have already begun the subtle "behavior modification" of their child through sex roles. Parents fantasize that their child will be "great"—will exceed their own capabilities, will magnify them in essence and act. The dream is inevitably cast in the male gender for the fantasy is that of the hero, and only males fit the mythic pattern of the hero. Unless consciously reversed, it is the boy baby that dominates the imagination of prospective parents.

Parents also relate differently to each child, depending on its sex. One father will relate to his daughter in a very different way than another father relates to his little girl, and so some will claim that there is no stereotypical programming involved. The crucial effect, however, is the fact that no matter how the father relates to his daughters, he will usually relate to his sons differently. Likewise, the mother. From the beginning, everything shouts *vive la difference* to the young child.

Ultimately, it is a destructive differentiation. It is the beginning of the "spell" cast on the young female, the onset of the gradual contraction of the world her imagination is allowed to live in, of the roles she is allowed to aspire to. She will be given dolls and "cooed" to more; her brother will have cars for toys and will enjoy more physical roughhouse. Later, when she asks for an erector set or a football, she might be coaxed into "wanting" something else. When she skins her knee or bumps her head, she will probably enjoy more soothing, protective assurances. She will be expected to be cleaner than little boys and certainly more manageable. She may, however, be more unmanageable *because of* these expectations. Scarlett O'Hara is a classic, if uncommon, example of this phenomenon in its adult form:

> I'm tired of everlastingly being unnatural and never doing anything I want to do. I'm tired of acting like I don't eat more than a bird and walking when I want to run, and saying I feel faint after a waltz, when I could dance for two days and never get tired. I'm

> tired of saying "how wonderful you are" to fool men who haven't got one-half the sense I've got, and I'm tired of pretending I don't know anything, so men can tell me things and feel important while they're doing it.[4]

Later on and with increasing intensity the cultural milieu and peer pressure will inhibit the little girl, discouraging her from being too assertive or too individualistic. She will learn the art of "fading into the wallpaper." Peer pressure and cultural attitudes will shape the little boy in the opposite direction, encouraging him to be competitive, aggressive and individualistic—even to the point of exhibitionism. In general, little boys receive much more opportunity for solving problems and modifying their environment.

The play activities of children reinforce these social expectations. Boys engage more often in physical activities—testing their limits constantly. Girls play, on the whole, more sedentary games—games that often prefigure the social role they will play in the future. Boys construct and contact, girls read and relate. And increasingly, children do neither—they watch TV, imitate and identify with the role models they see there.

Boys, however, are generally given much more exposure to team sports than girls. Through team sports they develop a capacity for "bonding" and a competitive resilience that is relatively lacking in girls. Among mature women this often manifests itself in an evident lack of capacity for female "bonding," in emotional inadequacy in competitive situations, in a tendency to overrelate to authority figures, in an unconscious fear of success and resentment of it in other women.

The assertiveness and independence factor in the young female is muted even further by the schooling years. Since most teachers at the elementary and high school level are white middle-class females, they tend to reinforce feminine or conforming behavior in the educational situation. Absorption and regurgitation of facts is commonly rewarded: questioning, objecting, arguing, conjecturing on alternative possibilities is, at best, uncultivated—at worst, discouraged and even punished. This atmosphere leaves most boys, who have been socialized to independent behavior since infancy, at a disadvantage. The schooling process inevitably categorizes females as "achievers" in their first twelve years of school. But with their entry into the collegiate arena, where debate and disagreement are exercised vigorously, women are at a disadvantage. Female deficiency in independent thinking is compounded by the emotional programming that has convinced the young woman, consciously or unconsciously, that demonstrating such skill is unfeminine. And, lest we forget, her teachers (who will be predominantly male in the better colleges and universities) have also been programmed with this expectation.

There's an old teacher's anecdote that demonstrates the truth of the matter very bluntly. It goes something like this:

> The difference between teaching an all-boys class and an all-girls class is that when you enter a class of boys and say "Good morning," half the hands shoot up demanding to know what you mean by "good," and the other half what you mean by "morning." When you say "Good morning" to a class of girls, they all write it down in their notebooks . . .

Of more critical significance is the fact that the developmental pattern of girls is less consistent than that of boys. Many young girls who exhibit active, creative and competitive traits in childhood drop these behavior patterns during adolescence and assume more feminine interests. At the same time, they show a rapid increase during early school years of withdrawal from challenging, problematic situations, and the IQ levels of achieving girls do not increase through the school years as do those of boys.

The "tomboy" phase, which often precedes puberty, is, for many young girls, the last eruption of individuated personality before the fall into "beauty" and the inevitable "sleep" of the female psyche. Very few, if any, boys ever wish they were girls. But many young girls share the fantasy of wanting to be boys. By middle childhood a preference for masculine roles appears in many young girls, along with varying degrees of disenchantment with the condition of being female. The tomboy temporarily transcends this condition and enjoys the best of both worlds—she is not measured by the same competitive peer-stature as her brothers, yet she enjoys the freedom of role experimentation, of aggression and engagement with reality, of daring and spontaneity. She gains a sense of self-determination, of comradeship, of control over her surroundings. For a brief moment, perhaps, in her life span, she is the warrior-maiden-adventurer—the archetypal androgyne. Soon, a part of her will be sacrificed. Psychologists have called it "animus," poets have called it "the left hand." Always, the metaphor signifies the same thing. It is a euphemism for the suppression of the capacity for self-actualization and transcendence. Dory Previn's song "Left Hand Lost" is a kind of lament for this lost wholeness, a dream of creative personhood:

> . . . sometimes
> i get so low so low
> sometimes
> i get so depressed
> as though i lost
> a part of me that loved me
> the part that knew me best . . .
> my right hand fills the china teacups
> and needlepoints with old maid aunts
> my right hand clings to rosary beads
> and waters dying plants
> but it's never painted a picture
> nor run for president
> my left hand
> might have done these things
> if its roots
> had not been bent
> a sculptor
> a poet
> it might have been
> instead of a useless thing
> to decorate with bangles and bracelets
> and my mother's wedding ring[5]

There is no experience comparable to the tomboy phase for prepubertal males. Boys are, in fact, not as free to express cross-sex preferences, and girls have much more latitude to indulge in a spectrum of male activities. Because the masculine role is dominant and associated with superior status, deviation from it by males is less tolerated. Girls, on the other hand, belong to a class of "outsiders," a group that has inferior status in the cultural paradigm. Like members of minority groups, they often show greater adeptness in role changes and are more psychologically free to experiment. While this elasticity diminishes greatly after puberty, nevertheless the fact that "it is more important for a boy to be all boy than for a girl to be all girl" remains constant throughout the life span.

By the same token, there is no male equivalent for "Daddy's little girl," and the female child is destined from her earliest years to learn how to exist for others. Although every little girl is endowed with her own motive and psychic force, she is soon equipped with two kinds of persona, to be tried on, occasionally worn, held in readiness for the future. She will specialize in one of the roles, or perhaps interchange both, later when she is a "woman." One persona is that of *the desirable object*. This role will school her in the art of cosmetic allurement, seductive mannerism and the sublimation of straightforward assertion. If she is well-disciplined in the role, it will leave her with a compulsive need for exclusive adulation. Her capacity for developing a healthy self-concept and strong peer relations will be crippled for life.

The second persona in the little girl's repertoire is that of the desire to *live for another*. This role will school her in self-forgetfulness, service and sacrifice, in nurturing rather than initiating behaviors. Above all, it will teach her to "sleep"—to wait, forever if necessary, for the expected *other* who will make her life meaningful and fulfilled. She will give up everything when the expected one comes, even the right of creating her own self. Whether it is a husband, a religion or a revolution, she is ready to live outside of herself, to abdicate from responsibility for herself in favor of something or someone else.

With the onset of puberty the feminine role becomes an imperative—the rehearsal is at an end, the real-life drama begins. The personae or masks that the young girl experimented with are now donned permanently. The creative, self-actualizing potential recedes gradually as the young woman is enveloped in preoccupations with her complexion, her popularity and her boyfriends (or lack of them). A dimension of her personality has been anesthetized, perhaps forever.

At this critical turning point in the young girl's life, the educational environment often exerts a crucial influence. Most junior and senior high schools are, in fact, mausoleums of the past. The whole process and organization of the school system tends to reinforce stereotypical norms and sex-role expectations, whether it is the teacher, the textbook, the curriculum or the peer stratification of the learning environment. Single-sex private schools can modify these effects somewhat, particularly in respect to the experience of "bonding" and achievement motivation, but a too premature and prolonged experience of this kind of environment can have diminishing returns—especially in terms of cross-sex socialization and academic competition. Moreover, a young girl might be at a disadvantage in merging from a female-dominated nurturing environment into the more impersonal milieu of social pluralism and corporate competition.

I learned the truth at seventeen
That love was meant for beauty queens
and high school girls with clear-skinned smiles
who married young, and then retired

The valentines I never knew
The Friday night charades of youth
were spent on one more beautiful
At seventeen, I learned the truth

—Janis Ian, "At Seventeen"

By the time they are seventeen, many young women have surrendered their ambitions to a growing need for affection, and their autonomy to an emotional dependence on the approval and good will of others. The spell is cast, and the promise of "beauty"—of being desirable—lulls the young woman into an existential limbo where everything is measured by the expectation of the one who is to come. Sleeping Beauty is not idle, however—she is busy living out the Pygmalion script (the male version of the myth), allowing herself to be sculpted, shaved, painted, plastered, pushed aside, pedestaled, pounded into a lifelike Galatea, the perfect fulfillment of a man's fantasies. At seventeen the young woman is well on her way to being a "formula female."

Giving advice to women has been one of the most constant industries in Western civilization. Whether it is the Church Fathers, modern psychiatrists, or Ann Landers, the message has been pretty much the same: Women are "different" (usually meaning "inferior") and they must accept the "role" that God and Nature intended (usually meaning what *men* would prefer). Advice literature boomed in America after the Revolutionary War, when industrialization and rampant capitalism aggravated the division of roles between men and women and created an impassable abyss between domestic and public life, between the home and the marketplace.

Most of the popular advice books written for women (by men) were designed to confirm and console them in the acceptance of their special "sphere," a function that excluded worldly achievements, assertive behavior, initiative and autonomy on the part of women. Like Sleeping Beauty, women were set apart from society by a "hedge," a range of interests that were identified as feminine: religion, the arts, homemaking, health and education. The literature of "the spheres" is still very much with us. It is the catalyst as well as the antidote for the condition of the contemporary woman. Anyone who has been programmed into help-needing, help-seeking dependency roles since birth, anyone who comes equipped with a built-in inferiority complex and naïve romantic expectations, in a real sense *needs* Ann Landers and Marabel Morgan.

The biggest consumers of advice are women. They soak it up like sponges: from newspaper columns and women's magazines, from TV commercials and soap operas, from best sellers and talk-shows, from ministers and priests, psychiatrists and gynecologists, from beauticians and galloping chefs and auto mechanics, from the housewife next door, from the mail man. Most women spend half a lifetime trying to measure up to someone's formula for the perfect woman. Some women are unfortunate enough to spend an entire lifetime at it. A few others make a living on it. Some die from it.

For the young girl, the formula is propagated in many ways, perhaps most blatantly by magazines like *Seventeen.* (Read by most girls when they are much younger.) The magazine, and the numerous *Seventeen* guides that complement it, exploit the adolescent girl's anxieties about being *a desirable object* and about the *hoped for other* (boyfriend, lover, etc.). Feelings and moods are frequently interpreted as functions of the same motif, repeated throughout the day—being noticed by "Number One Boy," getting a telephone call from "Number One Boy," seeing "Number One Boy" with another girl, daydreaming about Saturday night and whether he will ask her out. Not only emotional moods, but ethical judgments are locked into the "formula" anxieties. In a chapter on "The Question of Conscience" in one *Seventeen* guide, of the six sample situations demanding an ethical decision all except one deal directly or indirectly with the dating game or other formula imperatives.

The subversion of the whole educational experience is one byproduct of the formula propaganda and the advice industry. Witness chapters in *Seventeen* manuals like "School Is Where the Boys

Are," "Being a Good Flirt," "The Kind of Girl Boys Like," "Making Boy Talk," "You're Being Watched."[6] The chapter on giving parties is longer than the section on academic life. (In fairness, it must be noted that this is a book from 1965.)

Most of the advice is blatantly manipulative:

> Be seen where the boys are, at sports events, rallies, field practice.
>
> Take courses with labs. Working together in school can lead to dating together later.
>
> Go out for sports-slanted things like cheerleading, the marching band.
>
> Eat or walk alone sometimes. Solid packs of girls can scare off boys, while a lone lamb is often appealing.
>
> Smile and greet everyone. A friendly girl (you) is more fun to know.
>
> Carry something enormous: It may encourage masculine offers of help.
>
> Ask your favorite genius to help you with your homework. (Reward him with freshly baked cookies or brownies.)
>
> Offer to type his term paper. In return, ask him to proofread yours.
>
> Build his ego by asking him to explain a point he made in class.
>
> Ask his help with a confusing card catalogue or library index.
>
> Take extra-good notes—the kind he'll want to borrow.
>
> Compare grades with him—if you're sure his are at least as good as yours.
>
> Bring something complex to school: a camera, an exposure meter, a transistor radio. He'll enjoy instructing you in its use.
>
> Ask for advice on a gift for your dad or brother.
>
> Look your best always, and you'll always be ready if fortune (or a boy) looks your way.

The chapter on "The Language of Diplomacy" is little more than a catechism of dissimulation. And elsewhere, "The mythological Amazons and Valkyries took what they wanted by sheer female force, but real women have had to learn to mask their aggressiveness."[7]

The formula is summed up in a motif that repeats frequently in this kind of literature: concentrate on packaging yourself for consumption, but in conversation with men, "forget about yourself." What appears in print in *Seventeen* and the numerous advice columns for teenagers is a reflection of an ambience, a mental and emotional environment that envelopes the young girl from her earliest years and reaches its most destructive virulence in the high school years—the years of cheerleading, baton twirling, the popularity derby, going steady. It is the air that teenage girls breathe. The vampirish aspect of this programming is too often evident in the emotional investment that parents have in the process. At a recent baton-twirling conference on a Midwest campus, one zealous mother was observed at a drill practice yelling at her nine-year-old daughter to "Stick out your tits, honey!"

The formula is also the prescription for their middle-aged mothers, who are not exempt from the same imperatives. A classic reaffirmation of the double persona imposed on adult women can be found in Marabel Morgan's *Total Woman.* It is essentially a book of conversion, a manual of spiritual discipline for feminine backsliders (appropriately larded with scriptural injunctions) on fulfilling the role of: 1) *desirable object,* and 2) *living for another*. The book consciously undermines any idea that a woman might be man's equal and entitled to a self-fulfilling egalitarian relationship. The emphasis throughout is on "packaging" oneself for consumption, and the author's metaphors are occasionally as crass as her thesis:

> One of your husband's most basic needs is for you to be physically attractive to him. He loves your body; in fact he literally craves it. The outer shell of yours is what the real estate people call "curb appeal"—how the house looks from the outside. Is your curb appeal this week what it was five years ago?[8]

The objective of much of the advice in *Total Woman* seems to be to stroke the male ego enough to reduce him to a slobbering, adoring fool. In effect, the goal is adulation and creating the craving for it—not on relationship and communication (as between two autonomous persons), but on manipulation and dissimulation. Acceptance of the "total woman" ethic implies a mid-marriage "armistice," an implicit dialogue in which the husband says to the wife, "you be [on the surface] what I want you to be, and as a reward you can do anything you like on your own time."

Man: Don't disappoint my fantasies.
Woman: Don't disappoint my need for security, for being needed.

The scenario, in effect, exonerates both husband and wife from the need for growth and change. They have an arrangement, not a relationship.

The paralysis imposed on women by this kind of mass-produced formula has the ultimate effect of constructing a totally false persona and of suppressing the ego as well as the inmost self. The side of the personality that Gail Sheehy has described as the "merger self" overrides and dominates the "seeker self," and a sense of incompleteness becomes the characteristic experience of the female age group between puberty and marriage. These are the "desperate years" for young single women who work in offices, department stores, factories. They've been turned out of or excluded from the grazing pasture (college) where they would have easy access to an undiminished pool of available males. They have to survive, now, in a world of "closed dyads." The Saturday night date, the weekend at an army base, the engagement ring become the sole indications of progress. Maturity, spiritual growth and a sense of personal fulfillment are measured not by the young woman's internalized experience, but by her approximation to possession of an exclusive One. The longer she remains single, the more desperate she becomes, the more the "better-dead-than-unwed" paranoia increases. In all of this, the young woman abdicates from responsibility for self-actualization. She sees herself as someone that things will happen to, not as one who will make them happen. She has no conception of "autonomy" as a life-goal; she seeks only the state of "belonging to." From this, she will draw her identity and sustenance—the expected "kiss" of one who will awaken her from her dormant "sleep." What she does not realize at the time, is that the kiss of the first love will in all likelihood anesthetize her, fixate her at a level of development for years to come. The awakening may yet come, but it will be in mid-life. Sleeping Beauty is a time bomb.

> . . . What did you do with my soul?
> I gave it to others to hunt
> I gave it to our family to eat
>
> —"Words Between Man and Woman,"
> *The Three Marias: New Portuguese Letters*

Will a woman who remains single, or a woman who dedicates herself to a religious calling, escape the virus of "merging"? Not necessarily. The single woman can be trapped into the corporation consort role, the familiar "office wife"—who, perhaps, lives even more exclusively for her boss than the housewife. As for the religious woman, the risks of abdication are even greater: Her vows can be an excuse for relinquishing experience and ethical decisions, her community can provide a surrogate identity in place of her own.

Psychologically, Sleeping Beauty will inevitably show symptoms of her condition. These will tend to be of two varieties: "comatose" or "catatonic." Some women—the comatose—remain passive and submissive, consciously content with their role, but lacking a strong self-concept, dependent on someone or something outside of themselves for their identity and even their will to live. The possibility of shaping their existence, their environment, their self never occurs to them. They are accidental persons. In spite of their apparent stability and satisfaction, these women are often haunted by fears: fears of being left alone, fear of risking new encounters, fear of change, fear of conflict. In other women, the suppressed capacities may surface in more dramatic ways: in hyperactivity, in "clean freak" fetishes, in masochistic behaviors, in religious fanaticism, in hysteria, in possessiveness, in depression, in insomnia and nightmares, in headaches and peptic ulcers, in crying jags, in overeating. In some the "sleep" of the self takes on a concretely narcotic expression in alcoholism or a drug habit, or in just plain sleeping. Gabrielle Burton describes this syndrome:

> I read most of the time—in between sleeping. I wasn't working. I had stopped that when we were married, knowing it would undermine my husband's role as the PROVIDER. I lay around for nine months and ten days, waiting for my first fulfillment to come. I insisted that I loved being a housewife. Roger suggested once, in between my sobbings, that maybe I'd be happier if I went out and did something. What did he know? I knew with my extraordinary sensitivity that his ego would be shattered if I brought in a buck. Besides it would all fall into place when the baby was born.
>
> I slept inordinate amounts. It made me very guilty, but it also made the day go away and that was more important.
>
> Daytime sleeping is a form of suicide. Amazing numbers of women resort to it. Everybody knows it and pretends it is a necessity when raising small children and when a women tele-

phones another in the afternoon, she often says, "I hope I didn't wake you." It is common to hear, "Don't call between one and three. That's my naptime."[9]

Another of the most common afflictions of the formula female is consumerism. When the sense of self-worth is diminished, when sexuality is muted and functionalized, when access to power and decision-making experiences are minimal, women often compensate by a compulsive indulgence in acquisitive behavior. The "shopping syndrome," with all of its quasi-entrepreneurial activity—choices, opportunities (bargain days), mobility, plus the visual and social excitement of the marketplace—can be a substitute for creative work and the experience of power. It is one of the few public games that woman can play; it is stimulating and satisfying for the ego. In the exchange of money and objects there is a certain simulation of enterprise, of significant transcending acts of the will—and also, the sheer accumulation of things which provides a scaffolding for a weak self-concept. Possessions compensate for a low degree of self-actualization. Shopping is usually a tonic for a formula female.

But women have been victimized, too, by forces without as well as within. If women are more inclined to become shopping "junkies" than men, the blame can also be laid to advertising and commercialism which have systematically programmed and exploited the woman as consumer. In the public imagination as well as in her own private image of herself, woman has not been reflected as a creative producer but as the one who will consume and display what others (males) create and produce. This existential vacancy is readily filled with active consumption. It relieves anxiety and emptiness because what one *has* cannot be taken away. At the same time, it does not satisfy because it is incremental, requiring one to consume more and more to reach the same level of satisfaction.

There is a passage in Scott Fitzgerald's *Tender Is the Night* which offers a classic description and paradigm of the female consumer. Nicole, who has recently recovered from a breakdown, whose self-concept is fragile and in the process of dissolving again, emerges as a kind of emblem of the destructive forces—within and without—which inevitably entrap and exploit the American female.

> Nicole bought from a great list that ran two pages, and bought the things in the windows besides. Everything she liked that she couldn't possibly use herself, she bought as a present for a friend.

> She bought colored beads, folding beach cushions, artificial flowers, honey, a guest bed, bags, scarfs, love birds, miniatures for a doll's house and three yards of some new cloth the color of prawns. She bought a dozen bathing suits, a rubber alligator, a travelling chess set of gold and ivory, big linen handkerchiefs for Abe, two chamois leather jackets of kingfisher blue and burning bush from Hermes—bought all these things not a bit like a high-class courtesan buying underwear and jewels, which were after all professional equipment and insurance—but with an entirely different point of view. Nicole was the product of much ingenuity and toil. For her sake trains began their run at Chicago and traversed the round belly of the continent to California; chicle factories fumed and link belts grew link by link in factories; men mixed toothpaste in vats and drew mouthwash out of copper hogsheads; girls canned tomatoes quickly in August or worked rudely at the Five-and-Tens on Christmas Eve; half-breed Indians toiled on Brazilian coffee plantations and dreamers were muscled out of patent rights in new tractors—these were some of the people who gave a tithe to Nicole, and as the whole system swayed and thundered onward it lent a feverish bloom to such processes of hers as wholesale buying, like the flush of a fireman's face holding his post before a spreading blaze. She illustrated very simple principles, containing in herself her own doom . . .[10]

Nicole exemplifies, in another way, the ultimate form of female alienation—mental illness. The high incidence of schizophrenic symptoms among women, married women in particular, suggests that the problem is related to social role. As Chesler puts it, "Women more than men, and in greater numbers than their existence in the general population would predict, are involved in careers as psychiatric patients."[11] Our institutions are filled with and frequented by women in whom the delicate balance between an outer false self—or social role—and an inner true self has collapsed.

Thanks to some of the "anti-psychiatrists" like Laing and Szasz we can no longer classify these case histories simplistically as victims of "madness" or "insanity." The schizophrenic experience may in fact be a tactic, a strategy of escape from the "half life" of socially determined "normality." The inner self, under pressure and fear, retreats into isolation and fantasy, separating from the false self and the consequences of being embodied, situated and responsible. Because the schizophrenic withdrawal is often a response to personal invalidation, some psychologists have speculated that madness, whether it appears in women or in men is either the acting out of the devalued female role or the total or partial rejection of one's sex-role stereotype.

In the past the classic psychiatric treatment of this kind of mental illness in women has been the application of the "adjustment" model —a systematic programming of the patient to her role as supportive female and wife. Simone de Beauvoir has observed that, particularly in the case of female patients, psychiatry has substituted a concept of adjustment for the power of moral invention—in other words, a condition in place of a capacity. Woman has been denied the assertion of her transcendence by a mechanistic psychology which postulates her adaptation to a condition of alienation, submission to certain roles, processes, drives. When this sublimation fails to take place, she is regarded as abnormal—it is never suggested that perhaps the woman has *refused* to undergo the process of adaptation as a matter of choice.[12]

The failure of moral assertiveness in women has had obvious effects on feminine behavior. It has produced masked forms of aggression. Since overt aggressiveness is unacceptable in a woman, she may develop covert devices of verbal and emotional manipulation—guilt-producing mechanisms, habits of deception or evasion, ploys of helplessness, and even invalidism. Many of these syndromes have been attributed to woman's natural tendency to narcissism, but the self-preoccupation that this implies might better be described as a self-anxiety than a true self-centeredness. The formula female, conditioned to live for another, is obsessed with winning the acceptance and approval of the significant other. Her self-concern is focused on her impact on others rather than on her self.

Recent studies comparing "other-centered" women and "self-centered" women seem to bear out the pathological effect of this conditioning.[13] In one study, other-centered women—those who find it easy to be self-forgetting, self-effacing, altruistic, dedicated to a person or cause—generally exhibited a low self-concept. By comparison, the self-centered women—those who were less self-effacing, more concerned with self-determination and fulfilling personal goals —consistently revealed a higher self-concept and a more developed ethical personality. The other-centered woman is typically more exclusively devoted to a husband or family, but also makes more demands on those she lives with. Her expectations are generally higher and more pressurizing; her emotional dependency is high. She is more likely to play the "queen of the castle" role.

The self-centered woman, on the other hand, is more interested in a husband or partner who is kind to all. She expects less exclusive attention from him. She is generally less demanding in her expectations of all family members and less emotionally dependent on her husband and family. She is easier to live with and generally has a positive effect on others' sense of self-worth. If this seems paradoxical in the light of all that we have absorbed concerning "unselfishness" from our socialization, a correct understanding of the self-actualized personality resolves the dilemma. As one psychologist puts it, "The paradox of self-possessed people is that those who do not need the other can share best with the other."

Here we have reached the core of what personality as well as humanity means. Theologian Paul Tillich has described personality as being that which has power over itself. The power to do and to choose, the power to create one's own existence, the capacity for transcendence, is an obvious prerequisite for fully developed human personality. Self-determination is a prerequisite for the formation of an ethical capacity. Moral development is directly related to an individual's opportunity to make decisions in life, and this, in turn, is dependent upon the role one is permitted to play in society. Where social role relegates greater responsibility to an individual, there the moral development is generally the greatest (for good or ill). It is not power that corrupts, it is powerlessness.

For example, a cross-cultural study a few years ago[14] revealed that ethical capacity and maturity was generally higher in males, slightly lower in females of Anglo-American origins, and extremely low in females of underdeveloped cultures. Enterprise and decision-making have been the domain of the masculine; immanence the destiny of the feminine. It is the husband who goes beyond family interests to those of society, opening up new possibilities for his self through cooperation in the building of a collective future: he incarnates transcendence. Woman, by contrast, has been largely restricted to the role of continuing the species and caring for the home, condemned to the repetition of life rather than its transcendence, limited in the possibilities of the self, trapped in immanence. Woman has had an excuse for, and the luxury of, abdicating from responsibility for her own life, for remaining morally and existentially asleep.

> . . . many live in a quiet state of perdition . . . They live their lives outside of themselves, they vanish like shadows, their immortal soul is blown away, and they are not alarmed by the problem of its immortality, for they are already in a state of dissolution before they die.
>
> —Sören Kierkegaard, *Either/Or*

There is an inherent irony in this situation that makes it even more difficult for women to actually realize their condition. Centuries of dualism and misogyny have reinforced the conception of women as vessels of virtue as well as vice. Particularly in Western cultures, the temptress image has been complemented by the pedestal myth. With the onset of industrialization and the growing division between public and domestic life, the doctrine of "separate spheres" for men and women became a necessity. As men devoted themselves more exclusively to the marketplace, it was imperative that women specialize in those responsibilities and interests that their husbands had abdicated from. And so, woman became the guardian and protector of religious and cultural values, the chief model, educator and caretaker of the young, the spiritualized consort of her mate who necessarily devoted himself to Mammon. Woman's sphere thus contracted much from what it had been in more primitive times. Existentially, her life grew narrow, uneventful and even frivolous. The nineteenth-century image of woman as religious mentor and paragon of virtue created a social myth, an illusion about women's spiritual and ethical capacity.

Woman had become, in fact, a spiritual dwarf.

In consoling themselves and rationalizing their condition, women have embraced the notion of "being" as opposed to "doing" and have mapped out all sorts of female preserves to compensate for the exclusion from the real world. Acceptance of this condition, on the surface, may convey in many women the impression of maturity, self-acceptance and religious capacity. In reality, it is frequently a false spiritual imperialism appropriated by women to compensate for their moral deprivation.

From a Christian perspective, the haunting question which all of this suggests is whether or not the formula female is capable of redemption, of experiencing an awakening, of achieving transformation, and transcendence.

Among the more sophisticated expressions of the contemporary advice genre are several major contributions to what might be called "the literature of the life cycle." Erikson's paradigm of identity and the "Eight Ages of Man" has been a seminal influence. Gail Sheehy's recent *Passages* synthesizes the best from contemporary sociology of the life cycle and represents an empirical chronograph of characteristic human crises. Others offer an interpretation of human development on a more abstract plane: Robert Jay Lifton's paradigm of forms of symbolic immortality, of the Protean self and the death encounter represents a significant variation.

Disparate as they may seem, most of these paradigms have common roots in ancient myths about human growth. Two myths in particular seem to underlie many of literate culture's models of the life cycle: Ulysses and Oedipus Rex. They constitute, in a sense, the archetypes, the ur-images of our imagination of our own history. Freud, Erikson and all who have attempted to schematize the *rites de passage* of human development inevitably and implicitly echo these myths. Ulysses is the proto-myth of a whole pantheon of searcher-heroes whose transcendence, growth, is incarnated in the journey experience. Oedipus is the para-myth of those heroes whose progress is interpreted largely as a process of enlightenment, of what the Greeks called *anagnorisis*—passing from the state of unknowing to one of understanding. What is significant about both of these myths is that they are linear, historical and complete. Ulysses and Oedipus are different at the end of their respective journeys, they are transformed, they finish out their lives on a different plane of existence from where they began. Each has, in the pre-Christian sense, experienced a kind of *metanoia*. The traditional myths almost universally center around heroes who undergo a process similar to that of Ulysses or Oedipus. Significantly, females rarely, if ever, assume this role in the myths. Their involvement is peripheral and static, and even in cases where it is dynamic (Antigone, Medea), hardly ever is there any suggestion of transcendence to a new level of existence following the journey, the enlightenment or the encounter. Typically, they end as they begin, or they go mad, or they simply perish.

Mystical literature for centuries has also reflected this bifocal view of the spiritual process. Men have viewed their progress in the spiritual life as a journey, an ascent, metaphorically transcendent and existential. Women have more often resorted to the paradigm of the "inner room," the mansion, the castle—metaphorically a more static image, conveying the sense of immanence. The archetypal paradigms suggest that men transcend themselves and become "new" men, and that women on the other hand only learn better how to be themselves.

Inevitably, with the passing of time, mythology is translated into psychology. The heroic, androcentric bias of the traditional myths becomes the basis for models of the human psyche as well as the life cycle. Jung's theory, for example, of the "anima" and "animus" is a culture-bound concept rooted in a centuries-old rationalization of male dominance and extreme division of sexual roles. It is, perhaps, more symptomatic than analytical.

Likewise, Erikson's model presumes the male pattern to be the norm. Gail Sheehy has underscored how his concept of mid-life "generativity" misfits the situation of most women:

> All the male researchers into adult development agree with Erikson that the path to replenishment in midlife is through nurturing, teaching and serving others. Yet once again, the male life cycle is presented as the adult life cycle.
>
> Overlooked is the fact that serving others is what most women have been doing all along. What is the first half of the female life cycle about for the majority of women if not nurturing children, serving husbands and caring for others in volunteer work? If a young wife has any extra-familial career at all, it is more likely to be in teaching or nursing.
>
> It is not through more caregiving that a woman looks for a replenishment of purpose in the second half of her life.[15]

The myths of initiation suggest that another kind of model or "life map" might be more significant. The symbolic resonance of many of the ancient *rites de passage* remind us that there are rhythms that transcend the life cycle, that develop in harmony with it but are not inexorable. Philosophers, mystics and theologians have created paradigms that attempt to describe these rhythms, these metamorphoses of the spirit.

Kierkegaard, for one, proposes a threefold distinction between the aesthetic, ethical and religious modes of existence that may have special relevance for contemporary women. In this schema, the *aesthetic* life is that dimension of existence characterized by immersion in the immediate. Life is a succession of moments, a state of possibility—one has not yet made a positive choice of becoming a self. The aesthete is an "accidental man." Kierkegaard distinguishes a variety of expressions of this level of existence, drawing a radical contrast between its expression in men and women. If Don Juan is the archetypal male aesthete, his victims are archetypal female aesthetes. "To seduce all girls is the masculine expression of the feminine yearning to let herself be seduced once and with all her heart and soul." Thus, the absence of commitment to the self, the compulsion to "live for another," to be psychically annihilated and controlled by something beyond the self—common symptoms of female psychology—are the characteristics of the minimal level of spiritual existence. This level of existence is marked by illusion, since power over oneself has been given over to something outside oneself. The will-to-meaning is achieved at the expense of experience and the will-to-know. In this sense, Kierkegaard's paradigm of the aesthetic existence might be synonymous in effect, although not in expression, with an ascetic, repressed existence.[16]

In contrast to the aesthetic existence, the *ethical* life is based on a confidence in one's own power of choice, in one's capacity for righteousness and a certain self-sufficiency in undertaking the project of existence. "He who lives ethically has himself as his task." The ethical person has not duties outside himself but within himself. If there is a certain static fatalism to the aesthetic existence, the ethical life is dynamic. "The ethical individual so lives that he is constantly passing from one stage to the other." The ethical stage is marked by moral freedom and moral solitude. But the ethical life nevertheless fixes the spirit on finite existence; transition to another sphere of existence is yet possible. When the ethical stage brings man into contradiction with himself, it brings him to the edge of the transcendent.

In the third, *religious,* level of spiritual existence ethical man abandons his self-righteousness. Self-sufficiency gives way to self-transcendence, and the ethical stage culminates in a realization of how precariously man is bound to temporality and how little he achieves through personal endeavor. "The center moves from man to God." The religious existence is a synthesis of the temporal and the transcendent rooted in irony, humility and repentance. If the ethical life redeems the aesthetic, the religious life transfigures both.

A contemporary theologian, Paul Tillich, offers a paradigm similar to Kierkegaard's. His dialectical interpretation of cultural and religious history as a process of the interaction of heteronomy, autonomy and theonomy parallels Kierkegaard's tripartite model of ex-

[illegible] [illegible]llich's paradigm is no less applicable as a model for personal [illegible]ry, a kind of "life map" of the spirit. The analogy, and [illegible]t, to Kierkegaard is evident:

[illegible]my is a condition of being in which an alien law, one [illegible]s outside the self, religious or secular, is imposed on [illegible] 'It destroys the honesty of truth and the dignity of the moral personality . . . Its symbol is the 'terror' exercised by absolute churches or absolute states. . . . It kills our courage to act through the scruples of our anxiety-driven consciousness. And among those who take it most seriously, it kills faith and hope, and throws them into self-condemnation and despair." While the heteronomous authority originates outside the individual, it is imposed on the consciousness by the individual—as a result of the process of internalization and self-repression. Religious groups are often responsible for this internalization process: "The broken symbols of myth and cult press in from the outside." The life of the spirit is, in short, reduced to living for a code or concept extrinsic to the human personality.[17]

Autonomy is a condition of being that is "the obedience of the individual to the law of reason, which he finds in himself as a rational being." Autonomy "makes the inner life of the individual dependent upon itself." Its self-determination and independence, rightly comprehended, is not mere willfulness or a blind self-orientation. It is an acceptance of responsibility to "the law implied in the logos structure of mind and reality."[18]

Thus Tillich's notion of *heteronomy* and *autonomy* correspond analogously and in terms of the soul's orientation to itself and reality, to the *aesthetic* and *ethical* modes described by Kierkegaard.

Tillich's notion of *theonomy,* like Kierkegaard's concept of the religious existence, is a synthesis and equilibrium sustained between the tendency to self-sufficiency and to self-transcendence. It is "autonomous reason united to its own depth," to the ground of its existence, God. Human relations and personal fulfillment are not surrendered to the destruction of the will-to-power or libido, and at the same time they are not sacrificed to social, ecclesiastical or political norms.[19]

Among contemporary theories of ethical and religious development, Jim Fowler and Sam Keen's "life maps"[20] are analogous to the philosophical paradigms of Kierkegaard and Tillich. Fowler has integrated the work of the structural developmentalists Piaget and

Kohlberg in a comprehensive outline of life stages that corresponds to patterns of ethical maturation and faith development. The Kohlbergian stages of preconventional, heteronomous morality and conventional, interpersonal conformity, give way to a postconventional, autonomous ethical capacity and an ultimate loyalty to being. Fowler parallels the Kohlberg model to the stages of an emerging religious sense, grounded in cognitive symbolization. Sam Keen makes explicit use of Tillich's heteronomy/autonomy/theonomy paradigm in his scheme of personality-character construction. His models of the "outlaw" and the "sage" provide especially vivid archetypes for understanding the autonomous and theonomous stages of development.

The struggle—and, all too often, failure—of women to achieve ethical autonomy, has been the theme of the most significant fiction about women. As might be expected, such works are not numerous, but the few that we have are overwhelming testimony to what, for the most part, has been an agonizing, inarticulate struggle. Kate Chopin's *The Awakening*[21] documents the transformation of a genteel Calvinistic Southern lady from a submissive, repressed consort into a woman of passion and decision.

Edna's progress in achieving ethical autonomy is vividly charted in Chopin's portrait of a succession of dining scenes. At first, Edna cannot bear to finish her food when her husband walks out of the dining room in a snit. Her emotional dependence on his presence and approval is overwhelming. In her transitional stage, Edna forces herself to stay at the table and finish her food alone, in spite of his disapproval of her. Finally, in the later scenes of the novel she *chooses* to dine alone, and finds enjoyment and personal satisfaction in the experience. In a final act of social independence she dares to take a drink alone—first beer, then brandy.

Her rebellious seizure of autonomy is reflected also in her progressive adjustment of her living situation and daily schedule. Her first feeble attempt to emerge "on her own" is an excursion with friends to Mass across the bay—the exodus ends appropriately in a faint and emotional exhaustion. Later, she abandons the compulsory visiting days and begins to indulge in her own private excursions (rather bold behavior in the prim New Orleans culture of the turn of the century). Finally, she abandons her home and moves to her own apartment in an act of complete domestic and social defiance.

Chopin seems to be portraying a woman who has—at least, intermittently—achieved a capacity for ethical existence. While she does k to heteronomous behavior, nevertheless, her newly stincts for the aesthetic-sensual life lead her to a moral ch she resolves by suicide.

enina makes the same choice. In fact, few fictional her- ble to progress farther than these rudimentary stages of nique among many works featuring a female protago- nist, No rize winner Sigrid Undset's novel *Kristin Lavransdatter* portrays the life span of a woman with unusual completeness and density. The tripartite division of the novel as well as the experiential content described in each—*The Bridal Wreath, The Mistress of Husaby*, and *The Cross*—seem to echo the Kierkegaardian paradigm of the spiritual life. Indeed, Kristin reaches the threshold of transcendence in her short but full life, and passes over. She wrests ethical autonomy from an ineffectual, vain-glorious husband, and in the end redeems the consequences of her own blind self-will in her final days of solitary, moral heroism under humiliation and holocaust. Sigrid Undset's fiction captures the faith dimension of a woman who has come full circle:

> Never, it seemed to her, had she prayed to God for aught else than that He might grant her her own will. And she had got always what she wished—most. And now she sat here with a bruised spirit—not because she had sinned against God, but because she was miscontent that it had been granted her to follow the devices of her own heart to the journey's end.
>
> She had not come to God with her garland, nor with her sins and her sorrows—not so long as the world still held a drop of sweetness to mix in her cup. But she came now, now she had learned that the world is like a tavern—where he who has naught more to spend from is cast out at the door.[22]

> In the end, what difference can my absence from this world make to you, if all I gave you was my absence from myself . . .
>
> —"Monica," *The Three Marias: New Portuguese Letters*

Applying the paradigms of Kierkegaard and Tillich to the present condition of women suggests at least two critical questions:

1) Are women fixated at the first level of spiritual existence?

Have they achieved a certain "piety" that resembles the "ascetic," "seducible" variation of Kierkegaard's aesthete? And is this the cruelest seduction of all—to believe that one is religious when one has yet to acquire power over one's life?

Kierkegaard, in particular, emphasizes the critical nature of the ethical stage of existence—it cannot be avoided or omitted, it must be patiently traversed if one is finally to reach the threshold of religious existence. In one of his dialogues, Kierkegaard (in the persona of Judge Wilhelm) advises against a too premature entry into the religious stage.

No doubt the exigencies of many women's lives force them out of the heteronomous stage into an ethical existence, but all too many seem trapped unconsciously in a kind of aesthetic religiosity or reflex moralism. In this respect, as Peggy Way has observed, the Church has often become a "hiding place from woman's wholeness." The ancient question has an alarming relevance today: Can woman be saved? Can woman achieve true religious capacity?

2) A second critical question that these paradigms suggest is whether many of the crises currently emerging in male/female relationships and in family life are, in fact, symptomatic of woman's need for ethical autonomy and her struggle to achieve it. If so, what many look upon as the disintegration of "feminine" identity should rather be viewed as a moral imperative. What for men is a given, a self-transcending capacity imbued by socialization and cultural conditioning, is for women a quality that must be acquired, seized—painfully and often traumatically—sometimes very late in life. The contemporary migration of women into the marketplace suggests that meaningful work may have a significant effect on the achievement of ethical autonomy.

Finally, the Christian life calls everyone to a higher existence, to a faith that promises personal growth and transcendence, and at the same time demands the acceptance of suffering and diminishment. It is the enemy of complacency; it requires continuous conversion. The "life maps" of Kierkegaard and Tillich, in a sense, must be lived through again and again: Spiritual maturity is somehow a function of their dialectical relationship. To the extent that a woman's life does not engage this dialectic, she is doomed to be a spiritual dwarf.

The ultimate laws of the Christian life stand in contradiction to the image of the formula female:

"Love your neighbor as yourself."

"Let us not love in word or speech, but in deed and in truth."

One cannot love another until one has properly loved oneself. One cannot love others or God unless one has power over oneself, the power to choose and act. A sense of self-worth and a sense of self-creation are fundamental to spiritual maturity.

The kiss that Sleeping Beauty waits for is not that of any Prince, but the embrace of her own being.

the legend

Snow White . . . sent out by a jealous stepmother to perish, surrounds herself with safe, "small" men, each with a flaw. She waits and wishes to be found and rescued.

—D. Jongeward, D. Scott, *Women as Winners*[1]

These fairy-tale mothers are mythological female figures. They define for us the female character and delineate it possibilities. When she is good, she is soon dead. In fact, when she is good, she is so passive in life that death must be only more of the same. Here we discover the cardinal principle of sexist ontology—the only good woman is a dead woman. When she is bad she lives, or when she lives she is bad. She has one real function, motherhood. In that function, because it is active, she is characterized by overwhelming malice, devouring greed, uncontainable avarice. She is ruthless, brutal, ambitious, a danger to children and other living things. Whether called mother, queen, stepmother, or wicked witch, she is the wicked witch, the content of nightmare, the source of terror.

—Andrea Dworkin, *Woman Hating*[2]

The story of Snow White warns of the evil consequences of narcissism for both parent and child. Snow White's narcissism nearly undoes her as she gives in twice to the disguised queen's enticements to make her look more beautiful, while the queen is destroyed by her own narcissism.

—Bruno Bettelheim, *The Uses of Enchantment*[3]

One of our earliest imaginative companions is Snow White. As young girls we identify with her, perhaps more than with any other fairy-tale heroine. The tale is universal; variants appear in almost every language and culture. The story has a certain primacy in the reservoir of fantasy that is our heritage, no doubt because it is a metaphor of the most fundamental relation in human experience—the mother-daughter connection.

Snow White, like all metaphors, is both a program for exploring experience and a means of interpreting, explaining it. Existence brings with it a double jeopardy: Without an early and intimate relation to a mother figure, we can have no identity, no sense of our "self." Yet there is always the risk of an inherent destructiveness in the relation, a destructiveness that can cripple and deform the very "self" that it creates. The wicked stepmother is the invention of our fear:

> The myth of the stepmother is the obverse of the myth of the mother, although stepmothers are no better and no worse than mothers; in fact, since the stepmother frequently enters the child's experience later than in infancy, she cannot inflict the critical trauma the infant suffers at the hands of the mother. It follows, then, that the universal abuse of the stepmother is a way of providing a scapegoat for our fear and hatred of the mother.[4]

If the wicked stepmother is the central experiential element in the tale of Snow White, the truth-telling mirror is the most symbolic. It is an icon of the narcissism and envy that constitute the emotional center of the tale. Many versions of the fairy tale begin with a queen's longing for a child, a daughter, a reflection of herself. The queen's wish is fulfilled, she dies, a stepmother intervenes—the image of the "bad" mother emerges out of the "good."

Several versions of the tale are more explicit in dramatizing the oedipal roots of the queen's jealousy. (For example, in Basile's *The Young Slave,* an early version, the cause of the [step]mother's jealousy is the real or imagined love of the [step]mother's husband for the young girl.) The more popular versions, however, leave these connotations of incest to the imagination. Moreover, the dialectic of narcissism between the queen and the magic mirror is the dominant motive of the action. The wicked stepmother assaults her own soul, demanding reassurance of her desirability. The mirror—so like herself, so like a daughter—answers truthfully, but from a gradually changing perspective. Snow White becomes the object of a virulent, sadistic and masochistic envy. "Snow White shall die, even if it costs me my own life." Snow White is representative of the positive, life-asserting qualities that threaten the insecure, narcissistic personality. When the wicked stepmother devours what she believes to be Snow White's liver and lungs (vital organs), she recaptures a primitive cannibalistic expression of envy: the belief that one acquires the power and characteristics of what one eats. This fictional element is also symbolic of the mutilation fantasies often projected on the mother by her offspring, a psychological phenomenon familiar to child psychologists.

Snow White's sojourn with the dwarfs provides a period of growth as well as a time of testing. The condition of her apprenticeship is *work,* which she dutifully performs. She controls her impulses by restraining herself in sampling the dwarfs' table fare, by carefully choosing a "proper" bed. But her nature is ambivalent: "white as snow, red as blood." She is innocent, yet thirsty for life; she is eager to know, but also to feel. She struggles to escape her stepmother, but compulsively puts herself in her power again and again. She lets her in, despite the dwarfs' warnings and despite previous experience of her disguises and subterfuges. Snow White's own insecurity makes her vulnerable to the same temptations of narcissism that afflict her persecutor. Each temptation of the evil queen appeals to her vanity in a more intimate and essential way: first the scarf that binds her body, then the comb that "poisons" her head, and finally the apple—laden with death—which Snow White absorbs into the very heart of her being.

The dwarfs function as enigmatic witnesses of her gradual transformation. Many interpreters of the tale are fond of alluding to their "phallic" significance—they are "little men" who dig and probe the earth, mining it, "skillfully penetrating dark holes"—but this connotation seems of far less importance than a more traditional interpretation that associates them with the inhabitants of barrows and burial places, hence with "ancestral spirits." In the light of the denouement, they can be seen in this fairy tale as harbingers of death (for, in fact, they cannot revive her from the final poison). The dwarfs are fixed in their development; in contrast to Snow White, their lives are conflict-free, they are excluded from the process of transformation. Help for Snow White must come from beyond, from a transcendent force.

As in many mythic tales, an ambivalent fruit—the apple—is set before the heroine. She must choose whether to eat or forego the temptation. The risk of evil is inherent in the possibility of experience, whether that is sex, love, enterprise, knowledge, discovery. This broader generic meaning that lies behind the presentation of the apple is somewhat eclipsed by its pertinence to the fundamental structure of the mother-daughter relation. Mother shares the "apple" —female identity—with us. The apple is poisoned because the process is poisoned:

> I, who was never quite sure
> about being a girl, needed another
> life, another image to remind me.
>
> And this was my worst guilt; you could not cure
> nor soothe it. I made you to find me.
>
> —Anne Sexton, "The Double Image"[5]

In that poisoning, the "wickedness" we lay on mother is a projection of the sinister half of ourselves that we would like to repress. Yet so often our efforts to be what she is *not* confirm our inevitable similarity. As Bettelheim observes:

> The readiness with which Snow White repeatedly permits herself to be tempted by the stepmother, despite the warnings of the dwarfs, suggest how close the stepmother's temptations are to Snow White's inner desires.[6]

The relevance of the mother-daughter relation to the apple transaction is heightened by the association in religious iconography of the apple with the maternal breast, suggesting the inextricable relation between the mother-bond and human fallibility. Indeed, there is much in the tale of Snow White that is analogous to the traditional conception of original sin: "a condition of guilt, weakness, or debility found in human beings . . . prior to their own free option for good or evil. A state of being, not an act or its consequence."[7] The effect is the same: a deathlike sleep of the soul; a living death. The poison can only be dislodged by trauma and by the intervention of a transcendent presence.

If *Snow White and the Seven Dwarfs* dramatizes the negative aspect of the mother-daughter relation, another tale, *Snow White and Rose Red,* portrays a positive mother complex. Snow White, quiet and gentle, and Rose Red, extroverted and impulsive, are devoted daughters of a poor widow. Together they share an idyllic existence in an isolated cottage in a remote area—secluded, as the tale emphasizes by indirection, from the intrusion of any masculine presence, except for a friendly bear who visits now and then.

Snow White and Rose Red make several excursions into the forest. Each time they encounter an evil dwarf in some kind of difficulty. They are "full of pity" for the dwarf and each time aid in his rescue. In a final encounter, the friendly bear counteracts the sentimentalism of the two girls and kills the dwarf. His bearskin falls off, he is released from the spell cast by the dwarf, and is revealed as "a King's son." He and Snow White, and Rose Red and his brother, live happily ever after. The old mother lives "peacefully and happily with her children for many years."

The story may be interpreted as a parable of androgyny. The feminine "paradise" that the two girls share with their mother is portrayed as isolated from life, incomplete. The condition of fulfillment and happiness for the characters is that the girls will relinquish their feminine sentimentalism (the bear's act of aggression cancels this), and the prince must shed his "bearskin." (The origins of the work "berserk"—"bearshirt"—indicate that this connotes an excessive, masculine, warlike quality, a kind of machismo.) The tale suggests that this mutual transference of qualities is the key to humanization and social equilibrium.[8]

Both Snow White fairy tales—and there are numerous others—focus on the fundamental connection between women that is the precondition of their development into full personhood. The reality of our time in history requires that we reverse the pattern of the fairy tales—we must go back, restore and heal these female constellations in order to renew and integrate the suppressed masculine element. The Snow White motif becomes a metaphor for our aspiration to an "immaculate conception" of ourselves, exorcised of all crippling, life-denying effects of our socialization as women, of our destiny as daughters of our mothers.

TWO

Snow White and Her Shadow

IF the truth were told, most women would admit that they "prefer" the company of men.

A coffee break with the gal next door or in the next office is a necessary, even compulsive ritual. It is a kind of trading post for exchange of gossip, physical ailments, child-bearing practices, date debriefings, hang-ups, recipes and mutual support. But it is regarded as a secondary encounter, a dimension of life that somehow seems less important. After all, one's "real" life is lived with husbands and social partners—and *their* friends—with bosses and colleagues, with doctors and teachers, advisers and supervisors, most of whom are male. At least it seems that way, since most of the significant social roles in the average woman's network of relationships are filled by men. And, if the truth were told, being "one of the boys" is every woman's secret ambition.

Women have been subtlely prejudiced by the prevailing attitudes and mythology about the feminine condition to assume that relationships between women are bound to be trivial, inconstant, shallow, insincere. Women have come to believe that men are easier to get along with, more straightforward and loyal, and, above all, more interesting. Women have made themselves into pariahs among their own, behaving as they believe.

Cut off psychologically from her natural existential peers, deprived of basic training in "bonding," women are trapped into functioning as individual support systems for male enterprises and networks. They are needed, tolerated, used, much like bat boys or mascots on professional teams. The "groupie" image is symbolic of the female predicament: One establishes ephemeral female relationships in order to follow the rock star or team heroes. When female relationships are inconsequential, women are all the more vulnerable to male exploitation.

Thus, the radical estrangement at the root of woman's psyche is not alienation from the world of men, but from the friendship of women.

Where does it all begin? Who gives her the poisoned apple, who precipitates her escape to a world of psychic bondage to men?

We think back through our mothers if we are women.

—Virginia Woolf, *A Room of One's Own*

We come into the world as mirror images of our mother—destined to be not only her reflector, but also her silent inquisitor. The relationship between mother and daughter is the most intimate, most intense, most symbiotic and symmetrical bond known to humans. It is the great unexplored world, the unknown territory of the psyche. The arts as well as the sciences have probed, examined and dramatized every other relation: that of lovers, friends, brothers, fathers and sons, fathers and daughters, mothers and sons. But excursions into the emotional space inhabited by mothers/daughters have been rare and tenuous expressions.

For most middle-class daughters, the amount of time spent in contact with the mother is overwhelming. The infancy years, when we often enjoy the exclusive devotion of a non-working mother; the school years, when mother is chauffeur, maître d' and chaperone for all activities; the teenage years, when mother is chief social dispatcher and consumer representative (although this is usually a time when temporary snits and periods of estrangement are common); the college years and subsequent married life, when mother becomes an enormous resource of wisdom, and occasionally a babysitter and "summer camp" for the kids; the widowed or aging years, when a daughter becomes a companion and an important tie to a contracting world of activities and encounters; and, finally, in the weeks and months of illness, at the mother's deathbed, it is the daughter who is there, even in those lonely hours when her mother no longer knows that it is she, her daughter, who fluffs the pillow or soothes a fevered, pain-wracked body.

For many daughters, the time spent with a mother is a second lifetime. Walk through any department store, supermarket, subway, restaurant, resort, hospital—you will see them by the hundreds, mothers and daughters together. It is an all-absorbing relationship that generates enormous tensions and conflicts, yet, paradoxically, one that is the least expressed, the most taken for granted, the most impervious to interpretation. For some women, however, the time actually spent in contact with a mother is minimal or, worse yet, it may be an extremely negative experience. These less-fortunate daughters, however, do not escape the intense absorption of the mother relationship. In place of the actual presence of the mother (one who is perhaps dead, absent, or derelict) the child internalizes the *myth of the mother* even more desperately and passionately. The daughter may spend a lifetime seeking and projecting the lost mother or the "good" mother onto lovers, friends, mentors, even groups and institutions.

Because the prevailing social mythology of the American culture leads children to expect that they have a right to an exclusive mothering person who will offer unconditional love, meet all of their needs, and play certain stereotypical roles, anxiety and resentment are experienced when that expectation is not fulfilled. Mothers, too, are victimized by the mythology, for they are measured against an ideal fantasy that frustrates and confounds ordinary women. The overwhelming effect of the mythology is the perpetuation of extraordinary expectations on the part of children and inordinate guilt in their mothers. On the whole, American mothers are not confident in their mothering role and—faithful little mirrors that they are—children often confirm their feelings of inadequacy.

It is important not to underestimate the power of social mythology. The motherhood myth was initially one of the by-products of American independence and industrialization. As the division between home and the place of work widened and women's sphere contracted, it was imperative to insure that women would take up with fervor and dedication the domestic and socializing roles which men had totally abdicated from. Population was another obvious priority in a swiftly expanding industrial economy. And so, cultural mythology promoted the cult of "domesticity" and "republican motherhood."

One of the first important analyses and indictments of this pervasive and persistent mythology was Philip Wylie's *Generation of Vipers*. Published in 1942 in the midst of World War II, when there was a premium on patriotism and filial piety, Wylie observed that the "heroic mother" had to be cultivated in the public consciousness in wartime, or a mother's "natural pacifist" instincts might obstruct the progress of the war—she might refuse to give up her sons to slaughter. Wylie suggested that the more self-righteous a society is, the more optimistic and obstinate it is in its goals and ideology, the more the mother will be worshiped and the more society will expect of its mothers. His thesis seems to be confirmed by the evidence of Vietnam, when, in the late 1960s a severe disintegration of American self-righteousness was accompanied by a parallel disenchantment with the motherhood myth. Thus, the cult of the mother mostly waxes, and sometimes wanes, in our society in direct proportion to our faith in ourselves and our national projects. "Manifest destiny" could not have existed without it.

If this "imperial motherhood" has often been an acquiescence to the demands of a heroic cultural imperative, it has also been a gesture of protest and a kind of revenge. As a cross-cultural phenomenon, we can observe some interesting parallels in the experience of contemporary middle-class Mexican women. Unmarried Mexican middle-class women generally enjoy the freedom of economic and social emancipation. Once married, the life-style they have experienced as young women in the labor market is suddenly canceled. They are required to adapt to the highly traditional and restrictive role of the Mexican wife, a role that is aggravated by the prevailing mythology of machismo among Mexican husbands. The discontented Mexican wives seem to compensate for personal deprivation by investing all their ambitions and energies in the career of motherhood. The intensity of their dedication may also be a means of displacing male dominance in the family situation.

> The investigators observed that these *madres* almost literally tried to take possession of their children by conditioning their thinking, feeling, and behaving and by making certain that they would stay "faithful" to the mother. The mothers used affection—its conditional offering or withholding—as the major means of

> conditioning and controlling. This is the Mexican equivalent of the American mother's "conditional love" technique. The researchers concluded that, much like the American middle-class Mom, her Mexican counterpart aspires to "successful" motherhood because she feels she forfeited a meaningful career outside the home.[9]

No woman can escape the mythology. The American "formula female" must be converted overnight into a "good mother"—if the transformation doesn't "take," she is a failure. The process of motherhood becomes a perilous walk on a tightrope stretched between the myth and the reality. To keep their balance, mothers inevitably communicate with their children—especially their daughters—in an equivocal language.

Very early, a daughter intuits the double meaning in her mother's messages: "I'm your mother. I do everything out of love for you." ("Some things I do because it's expected. I sometimes resent these obligations because of what you did to my life.") "You're my daughter. I love my reflection in you." ("There are things in you I dislike, reflections of my own self-hatred and fears.") "I want you to love your body as I do." ("But I am uncomfortable with my own.") "I want you to be self-sufficient." ("But not ungrateful. I want you always to need me.") "I want you to be able to achieve something, to assert yourself." ("But I don't want you to be unfeminine.") "I want you to be more than I was able to be." ("But you can't have your cake and eat it too.")

And so the first "signs" that a daughter learns to read in her mother are signs of ambivalence about what it means to be a woman. She transmits to her daughter what one psychiatrist has described as "the fear of being a woman."

The female monopoly over early child care intensifies the mother-daughter relation. The primordial experience of absolute power for all children is located in the mother, in the experience of female will. Our first responses to pleasure and pain are associated with her, and thereafter, her shadow hovers over all our experiences of intimacy: those that are nurturing, and those that are destructive. It is she who structures our being to enjoy the security of symbiosis and to fear the trauma of separation.

And so, as in the fairy tales, we split our mother image in two: the nurturing "good mother" whom we think of as our real mother, and the destructive "bad mother" whom we associate with other women who are incapable of maternal love—the archetypal stepmother. It is an inverted perception, for the "good mother" is, in fact, an introjection of the myth, and the "bad mother" is a fantasized assessment of the limitations of a real mother, a projection of our own fears. This perhaps explains why psychiatric patients overwhelmingly represent the mother as "wicked" or why some "construct elaborate defenses against perceiving such feelings."[10]

Thus, the myth of the mother contributes to the creation of a woman who is a heteronomous personality, one determined largely by values and expectations that are imposed from without rather than derived from within. A woman who gives birth to a child long before she has given birth to herself faces the impossible task of raising an autonomous daughter.

Nevertheless, the symmetry between mother and daughter lends every woman a degree of determination (and false confidence) in shaping her daughter that her sons do not necessarily experience.

> Mom doesn't fuss much with her son, but she is constantly adjusting, fixing, trying to perfect this little female picture of herself in the same way she fiddles with her own never-perfect appearance.
>
> Like a puppet on a string. Mother feels entitled to manipulate her daughter because she, the mother, is a woman. She knows the way. She's the expert on women.[11]

Likeness produces a special tyranny (almost all the fairy tales that highlight a wicked stepmother involve a daughter, seldom a son). In self-defense, mother becomes a perfectionist in female socialization, a faithful interpreter of the traditional feminine role. Two messages in particular repeat most often (explicitly or implicitly): "no excess" and "no excelling." A mother moderates and limits her daughters; she will likely reverse this pattern with her sons. This moderating influence of mother over daughter is commonly observed in her efforts to curb excessive affection in the daughter. It begins in infancy: for boy infants the mother's affection and approval will be confirmed with a loving hug, a pat, a touch or some other physical expression. If a little girl infant performs the same action, she will often be rewarded only with a smile on her mother's lips, or a verbal compliment.

> The subtle deprivation of physical demonstrations of affection that little girls often suffer from their mothers makes women more vulnerable to fear and the loss of attachment; they were never sure of it to begin with. It makes women greedy to hold on even to men who treat them badly, more possessive and competitive for whatever crumbs of love may be available to them . . . The absence of physicality—which is the most direct communication of security and approval a mother can give an infant—means she will not be nearly as rich in autonomy and self-esteem.[12]

Male toddlers will be expected to "play with themselves," attempts at masturbation will be tolerated in them. In young girls any overt expressions of physicality—even curiosity—will usually be closely monitored; checked by the mother. And so, girls learn to be furtive and suspicious about their own bodies.

Later, when the daughter is old enough to understand compliments, a mother may ration her own expressions of praise and limit the degree of adulation the daughter will be allowed to accept or seek from others. Her mother's fear of excelling and of exhibitionistic behavior will "moderate" the young girl's budding vitality.

With her daughters, especially, the mother behaves like a mollusk. Alternately opening, inviting intimacy, affection and exploration; then closing abruptly, stringently, when the child demands or discovers too much. The mollusk tactic only increases the dependency of the daughter on the mother—she is teased and starved into a symbiotic attachment. She will be addicted to this kind of relationship all her life.

> A mother does not merely pass on the messages of her culture; she also passes on her responses to the messages she received from her mother. Thus, every transaction between mother and daughter is in a sense a transaction among three generations.
>
> —Signe Hammer, *Daughters & Mothers, Mothers & Daughters*

Mother and daughter are thus inextricably linked in a reciprocal self-reflection, two mirrors that constantly seek affirmation from each other but are often capable only of reflecting an ambivalence, a congenital insecurity of low self-esteem and ego denial.

Ironically, although women have often been labeled as "narcissistic," their self-preoccupation can be better described as self-anxiety rather than a true self-centeredness. Self-worth and a firmly anchored sense of identity are the result of an early narcissistic intimacy with a mothering person, a symbiosis that should lead to individuation and separation. Unfortunately in the mother-daughter relationship, this process is frequently attenuated. Instead of a healthy self-centeredness and resilient ego, the daughter is more likely to develop an intense self-preoccupation. This self-scrutiny is a neurotic narcissism, a compulsive, sustained observation of a false self created to fill the void in identity—not a secure centeredness in a spontaneous self. In its most acute form, this psychological vacuum can produce a schizophrenic personality. A more pedestrian and typical expression is the "formula female." She is likely to be a person who masks an inner self charged with hostility, fear, and envy, who fluctuates between extremes of vanity and self-deprecation.

And so, narcissism must be understood in a double sense. A healthy, primary narcissism implies an individuated self-centeredness. More often, however, narcissism implies the symptoms we have just described. For most women, it is a crucial obstacle in the development of full personhood.

The primordial contamination by both the myth and the reality of motherhood exacts a toll. Too often the symbiotic relation to the mother is merely transferred rather than outgrown. Too often the relationships of adulthood are not true encounters with the "other" but more a matter of switching mothers. The emotional responses of the daughter's arrested development play the same refrain over and over, like a phonograph needle stuck midway through a record.

The repetition syndrome is evident also in the familiar protests of daughters that they are "not like" their mothers. "Oh, no, I'm not at all like my mother. It was my father—my grandmother—who influenced me most." Denials, inevitably contradicted by the reality. Daughters invariably absorbing, repeating a mother's emotional life. Self-knowledge comes much too late:

> The older I get, the more of my mother I see in myself. The more opposite my life and my thinking grow from hers, the more of her I hear in my voice, see in my facial expression, feel in the

> emotional reactions I have come to recognize as my own. It is almost as if in extending myself, the circle closes into completion.[13]

Daughters are the primary heirs of a mother's psyche, and young women in the contemporary era are no exception. The "backlash" phenomenon is often evidence of a successful inoculation, in spite of the mother's verbal protestations of liberation. The daughter is likely to conform to the mother's unconscious feelings and responses rather than to her raised consciousness.

This may also explain the fear-of-success syndrome in exceptional women, and the tendency of achievement-oriented women to slip back into regressive roles after marriage. "Mother began to teach us how to be a woman and a wife long before dad came along to teach us how to be a success in the office."[14] It will take more than one generation to untie the mother-knot.

Likewise, the dramatic rise in teenaged pregnancies reveals compulsions that are not unrelated to the mother-daughter relationship. One recent task force report on teenage pregnancies indicates that the U.S. has one of the highest birth rates among adolescents in the world—58 births for every 1,000 females in the 15- to 19-year-old bracket. The sexual revolution is often blamed for these alarming statistics. Teenagers' explicit rationalizations often suggest other factors: "I wanted someone I could love and who would love me." "I wanted to have something of my very own." Below the surface lies another, more fundamental explanation: Many of these young girls are caught in the web of arrested symbiosis. They want to recapture with their own child the engulfing and/or aborted narcissism of the mother-bond, to experience themselves as objects of exclusive love. At the deepest level, their own self-esteem and sense of self-worth has been crippled, and the only compensation lies in repetition.

It is only in recent years that contemporary art has begun to probe the abysses of the mother-daughter relationship. A trickle of memoirs, novels, plays and films have dared to explore this uncharted territory. Mothers and daughters are invading the ego spaces of dramatic representation in a way that suggests it is the last psychic frontier. In understanding it better, we will understand ourselves better. The cinema, in particular, is an especially effective medium for mirroring the subtleties and nuances of what is going on between mothers and daughters, much of which is non-verbal.

The mythology still lingers, but a more ironic perspective is emerging—a demythologizing of both roles. Altman's surreal *Three Women* presents a matriarchal parody of the patriarchal family—perhaps more of a reflection of male fears about angry women and the disposability of men than a true reflection of female relationships. *The Turning Point* celebrated the "good mother," but also acknowledges the degree to which her motherhood has made her something less than she might have been and dramatizes her realization that her daughter needs more than one mother figure. *Autumn Sonata* focuses on the "bad mother," but with an ambiguity that marks it as a superb vehicle of complex human feelings. The bad mother is still portrayed, in this film, as the exclusive source of the child's unhappiness and character flaws—from the daughter Eva's point of view. The other point of view, painfully muted, is suppressed in the inarticulateness of the crippled, disease-ridden second daughter, Lena. The ritual of reciprocal torture enacted between Charlotte, the mother, and Eva, the daughter, silently witnessed by Lena, is a terrible testimony to the force of this primary relationship. The silence and immobility of the daughter Lena is symbolic of the contemporary struggle in which we pass dumbly through a painful exorcism of the myth of motherhood, longing for a time when mothers and daughters need not blame each other for so much because they have not needed each other so much.

> Who do we kill, which image in the mirror, the mother, ourself, our daughter????? Am I my mother, or my daughter?
>
> —Anne Sexton, *Letters*

Mother is the first mirror we gaze into in search of self-affirmation. The reflection is often ambivalent and distorted, and so our search for other mirrors—other women—is hesitant and uncertain. Whether we seek them as soulmates or role models, we are more likely to cling to them as life rafts than we are to trust our own buoyancy and ego strength. We have noted the more affective and effective nurturance that mothers generally give to boy infants by comparison with girls. This deprivation tends to be characteristic of the relations of women in general. Phyllis Chesler observes:

> Female children are quite literally starved for matrimony: not for marriage, but for physical nurturance and a legacy of power and humanity from adults of their own sex ("mothers").[15]

And so inevitably, we expect too much—or too little—of our relationships with other women. The effects of female socialization considerably diminish our capacity for authentic sisterhood.

In recent years a great deal has been said about the need for female "bonding." It is assumed that males have mastered the art, and that women haven't—largely because they haven't had the same opportunities. Yet, like men, since they were three or four, and certainly since age six, most of their play experience has been with same-sex peers. In fact, with the exception of dating, courtship and marriage, a woman's world—like that of most men—is a sex-segregated world.

So it cannot be claimed that society—at least in the formative years—isolates women from each other. Yet males "bond," women do not. Obviously the phenomenon has a connection with the qualitative nature of the shared experience. Men generally have experienced more team sports in growing up or at least the "team" ambience; and when they are grown up, they usually engage in more problem-solving, world-making enterprises than women. And so, clearly, the significance of the project that is shared is more critical than the degree of intimacy. (Women exchange "intimacies" but do not "bond.")

But women should be ambitious for more than male experience has provided thus far in our social relations. The myth of male bonding is as overrated as the myth of motherhood, when we compare the reality with the illusion. Bonding, for most men, provides a certain superficial cement and support function in their lives, but it does not produce friendship or intimacy. Men gather to talk shop, make business deals, drink, play golf—but not to be intimate, not for self-revelation:

> Men are particularly comfortable seeing each other in groups. The group situation defuses any possible assumptions about the intensity of feeling between particular men and provides the safety of numbers—"All the guys are here." It makes personal communication, which requires a level of trust and mutual understanding not generally shared by all members of a group, more

> difficult and offers an excuse for avoiding this dangerous territory. And it provides what is most sought after in men's friendships: mutual reassurance of masculinity.[16]

The combat "buddies" of World War II, the "cop couples" of popular TV shows, and the Paul Newman-Robert Redford syndrome in films reinforce the myth. Close analysis often reveals the ephemeral and shallow quality of these relationships. For example, during the last war English observers were confused by the apparent contradiction between American soldiers' regard for the "buddy," and the results of detailed inquiry that showed how transitory these buddy relationships really were.[17]

By contrast, women are not so comfortable in groups—chiefly because it confirms and accentuates their identity as females, a class excluded from the dominant caste in our society. In part, these feelings are introjections of a traditional male paranoia about women in groups. Aristophanes treated the projection humorously in *Lysistrata.* Early American conduct manuals cautioned men against allowing their wives to associate too much with their female peers, lest the "neighborhood squadrons of she-commanders" might encroach on their "natural sovereignty" as husbands. Others with less of a sense of irony or righteousness have treated the problem with sadistic vengeance in purging "witches" and other harbingers of female energy. In a typical business office today, a bevy of secretaries excites no notice. But half a dozen women junior executives having lunch together is likely to conjure up "conspiracy" in the minds of many men. Likewise, on a university campus, if one sees a group of men together it does not penetrate the consciousness at all. Nor does a group of female undergraduates. But a group of women faculty: How the comments do fly! How the plots do multiply!

What is happening, of course, is that a dominant caste is reacting to a threat to their established sway. This perhaps explains why men who can tolerate male homosexual pairings are nevertheless outraged by the idea of lesbian couples. It is perceived as an act of social anarchy.

Women can be forgiven for their instinctive uneasiness in all-female groups. Unless they are somewhat isolated from the real world (as with convents and girls' schools), they are bound to experience negative projections from the surrounding social texture. So women are more comfortable in intimate, private relationships. And yet, they are no more capable of true friendship than their male peers.

Friendship, in the true sense of the word, is perhaps the most singularly uncultivated capacity in American social relations. A relationship between equals, whether of the same sex or not, that implies intimacy, loyalty, sharing that is unconditional and unselfish—outside of marriage—is a rarity in our culture.

Anthropologists have described the phenomenon of "archetypal dyads" specific to individual cultures and the influence these have in the construction of social reality: Europe, with its father-son hegemony, Africa with its brother-brother, tribal primacy. In America the dominant archetypal relation is the romantic couple, accentuated by the myth of the New World, the Edenic beginning. The romantic dyad exerts a powerful, inexorable influence on all relations within the culture and implicitly denies the validity of other constellations. Inevitably, the significant "other" is viewed as a potential sexual partner. Hence, there has never been a well-defined social role in our society for the *friend* of the opposite sex, particularly for married persons. The tyranny of the "romantic dyad" is such that it tends—in our society—to invest all relations with a sexual ambience. Thus, the disproportionate fear, in same-sex relations, of allowing the relationship to become too personal, too homophilic. The fear is symptomatic of a culture permeated by neurotic narcissism, so often characterized by genitalization, misogyny, anality and homosexuality. The American culture, on the whole, is not a hospitable climate for fostering authentic friendship, either between men and women, or between persons of the same sex.

If society is hostile to friendship, women themselves are handicapped by conformity to the feminine sex role. The formula female is not likely to create lasting friendships. Her orientation to a single exclusive relationship and her need to invest all her emotional energy in it, makes it difficult for her to sustain intense love for more than one person at a time. Conversely, the idea that the loved one might also love someone else with equal intensity is extremely threatening. The pattern is visible in young girls who would rather play only with their "best girlfriend," to the exclusion of the group. It is a rehearsal for the ultimate "One," the exclusive, single relationship that supposedly will bring complete fulfillment. Nothing else, no other relationship really matters.

The conventional female role fixes a woman's priorities in relationships. Friendship with a woman is sustained only when it does not conflict with or threaten the important male relationship. Every woman knows what it is to be "ditched" of an evening by a female friend, when that significant "One" phones and asks her out.

The other-centeredness of the conventional female role, as we have noted before, diminishes the capacity for authentic peer friendships by making women susceptible to indulging in control mechanisms: "Her overidentification with the other person means she cannot tolerate behavior different from her own. She imposes a heavy load of shame and guilt if the other fails to do as she says."[18] The conventional female role also conditions women to need admiring inferiors and approving superiors. Women probably have less experience in, and less motivation, for relating to others as peers, comrades, colleagues and friends. Their need for symbiotic relationships and someone to shore up their fragile egos explains the vague (and sometimes almost hysterical) feeling that many women experience when confronted with silence in a conversation or a prolonged period of solitude. Needless to say, it explains, too, why many women fear new social situations and are less inclined to "explore" on their own. Mobility is often an index of autonomy.

The repression of overt behavior in women has also handicapped their capacity for friendship by conditioning them to passive aggressive behavior. Since overt assertiveness is less acceptable in a woman, she develops covert devices of verbal and emotional manipulation. Guilt-producing mechanisms, or even, a simple gesture like a prolonged stare—which may be a substitute for a punch in the mouth! She may develop habits of deception or evasion, or ploys of helplessness, even invalidism. She may say "yes" when she means "no," fake what she doesn't feel. She may share intimacies and gossip with another woman, but she lacks the spontaneity, directness and inner security that authentic friendship requires. Her self has not yet shed the layers of hiddenness, the masks, the false faces, the "shut-upness" described by Kierkegaard as "the state of being in sin." She lacks what he calls the fundamental quality of the spiritually whole person: *transparency*.[19]

The "shut-upness" is not only psychological, but also physical. Women are, on the whole, fearful and insecure where their bodies are concerned—even ashamed of their bodies. In part an introjection of social attitudes that denigrate female anatomy, and in part a result of maternal deprivation-guilt mechanisms, women are afraid of being "physical." They are conditioned to experience physicality—whether violent, destructive or pleasurable only when it is instigated by a male. Moreover, this phobia, along with their exclusion from team sports and athletics as children, deprives women of the healthy narcissistic pleasure of physical equilibrium and control of environment that is cultivated in males. The physical energies of women have largely been channeled into nurturant expressions or into seductive sexuality. Thus, women tend to avoid or disparage assertive physicality in other women.

Physical inhibition is another obstacle to the "transparency" required for authenticity and friendship. It also produces a vulnerability to commercial exploitation. One reason the evil stepmother can tempt Snow White so easily is Snow White's insecurity—she, too, is worried about "who is the fairest of them all." She succumbs, not to temptations of Promethean hubris, but to the vain trifles of the feminine mask.

> I asked her cruelly and brutally, as Henry might have asked, "Do you love women? Have you faced your impulses towards women?"
>
> She answered me so quietly ". . . I have faced my feelings. I am fully aware of them. But I have never found anyone I wanted to live them out with, so far. I am not sure what it is I want to live out."
>
> —Anaïs Nin, *Diary*

If there is any one of the traditional "Seven Deadly Sins" that is most representative of the obstacles to female autonomy it is undoubtedly the sin of Envy. The green-eyed monster is particularly characteristic of the relations between women—not in the petty sense that popular belief assumes, but in a deeper, much more fundamental way.

Simone de Beauvoir has described the problem of friendship among women:

> Women's fellow feeling rarely rises to genuine friendship, however. Women feel their solidarity more spontaneously than men; but within this solidarity the transcendence of each does not go out toward the others, for they all face together toward the mas-

> culine world, whose values they wish to monopolize each for herself. Their relations are not constructed on their individualities, but immediately experienced in generality; and from this arises at once our element of hostility . . . Women's mutual understanding comes from the fact that they identify themselves with each other; but for the same reason each is against the others.[20]

Woman is the archetypal outsider. Her psychic existence is, consciously or unconsciously, similar to the experience of many ethnic subcultures and racial minorities—persons whose existence is dominated by an overriding sense of cultural distance and who, therefore, live by virtue of their culturally accidental lives a symbolic and vicarious existence. Anthropologists have observed that one of the most crucial factors inhibiting vertical mobility in ethnically stratified societies is the problem of envy. Among many Hispanic subcultures, for example, advancement and success is equated with betrayal of the group, a sell-out to the "Anglos." Thus, the more gifted among Spanish-speaking people are often reluctant to take a leading role because of the resentment and ostracism it may engender. The majority, in fact, may keep their distance from potential leaders, and the ghetto perpetuates itself. This tendency can also be observed in the black community. Likewise, among primitive tribal families, individual excellence may be greeted with displeasure and envy. There is a characteristic aversion to the emergence of strong leadership.[21] This phenomenon explains the slow rate of cultural growth because it fosters resistance to innovation.

One should not be surprised, therefore, at the strength of the backlash in the wake of the feminist movement. The situation is analogous; it is an overwhelming expression of envy. It contains the recognizable features of its anatomy: fear of another's success, self-pity, blind trust in past security, identification with a clearly defined subordinate social role. As with subcultures and primitive peoples, it is a reactionary response to anyone capable of creating change.

"Ubiquitous envy, fear of it and those who harbor it, cuts off such people from any kind of communal action directed toward the future."[22] Within the women's movement itself, a great deal of this fear remains to be exorcised. When women in groups do succeed in overcoming this indigenous trait, they begin to have an impact on society.

If envy is a political fact of life for most women, it is also a personal problem for many. Adrian Van Kaam sees it as the most fundamental and crucial index of personality. One is either an "original" personality or an "envious" personality. "Originality" is simply another definition of self-actualization, self-centeredness, autonomy. The original person has a strong self-concept, motivation, decisiveness, creativity. The original person is not crippled by self-consciousness or fear, by compulsion from within or obstacles from without. They have an inherent or acquired ability to work, to play, to enjoy, to laugh, to fantasize, to loaf, to be serious, to be spontaneous —to be themselves.

The envious personality, as might be expected, is usually the opposite. Personally insecure, other-centered, driven by heteronomous motives and self-anxiety, the envious person is both victim and victimizer. The crucial element in envy is the instinct to "level," to equalize. "The envious man does not so much want to have what is possessed by others as yearn for a state of affairs in which no one would enjoy the coveted object or style of life." Envy is destructive. If the envious person does not succeed in "leveling" the object of the envy, the hostility will likely be turned on the self. "The envious man is perfectly prepared to injure himself if by doing so he can injure or hurt the object of his envy. Many criminal acts, in some cases perhaps even suicide, become more comprehensible if this possibility is recognized."[23]

To the extent that women are cut off from self-actualization and transcendence, they are destined to be envious. Among the symptoms associated with the envious personality are many that have been regarded as "typical" of the feminine condition. They are, rather, the symptoms of deprivation of the means to full humanness, originality, wholeness.

For example, while envious persons often indulge in aggressive destructive tactics such as gossip, slander, or "informing" that devalues the object of their envy, they are just as likely to indulge in behaviors that devalue themselves. Expressions of self-disparagement—"I'm too emotional to handle this," "I just melt when I'm criticized," "I can't think of anything to say," "I couldn't do what she does"—may be indications of envy. Depression, low-energy patterns and passivity are also characteristic escapes for the envious personality. "I can't do it, therefore I won't do anything." Inertia and envy are sisters. Self-pity and masochism are perhaps its most extreme expressions.

The envious person can also find compensation in fantasies of accumulation or emulation. Envious men may fantasize about celebrity, wealth, omnipotence; they may make impulsive career changes or drop out of school. For women, the fantasies are more likely to be connected with attractiveness and consumption, the withdrawals may be addictions. The envious person often directs his/her frustrated ambition toward a high level of consumption of goods that cannot easily be shared. One chooses to *have* instead of to *be*. This is not to say that only the affluent are envious. Consumption is relative. Monks, nuns, even the very poor and propertyless are just as likely to substitute consumptive having for creative being.

Envy is, of course, the most serious obstacle to friendship and bonding. In its worst form, it ignores, denies the existence of the other. "I could forgive you anything, except that you are, and what you are; except that I am not what you are." The habit of envy feeds on itself; the envious person constantly interacts with others in such a way that the envy cannot be assuaged. Kindness may even make it worse. The perception of the other is distorted; squinting, the envious person goes on perpetually reinfecting herself/himself with the disease.[24]

Envy develops among equals or among those who are almost equal. It is a phenomenon of social proximity. Hence, the housewife who depends on the woman next door for companionship and solace may—at the same time—be extremely envious of her. Real friendship between the two may be impossible, because their respective insecurity makes them essentially envious personalities. The failure to love those who are close by may, paradoxically, result in a displaced love for those who are distant. Involvement in abstract causes, social justice movements and volunteerism can sometimes be the result of an inability to establish authentic friendship with those who are nearest—in one's family, neighborhood, office or social peers.

For many women, life becomes a seesaw, a balancing off of one's own envious impulses against the fear of provoking another's envy. This is perhaps the most fundamental quality of the heteronomous life. Much that has been said about "the fear of success" in women might better be described as the "guilt of being unequal." Even in a steno pool, the rapid speed of one typist will arouse in her slower coworkers a sense of guilt which may paralyze their efforts to improve. What is even more tragic is the probability that it may cause the speedy typist to feel guilty for her ability to excel, to moderate her efforts or perform self-punishing gestures to win the others' forgiveness. Envy-avoidance is as destructive of female autonomy as envy itself. It is especially characteristic of groups in which large numbers of women are present: offices, schools, religious organizations. The fear of overexposing one's originality may finally cripple it. Again, the dilemma of Snow White:

> When the tactics of envy endanger the effectiveness of my life and work, I should take them seriously and deal with them wisely. I may be tempted to give up resistance simply because I want so much to be in with the gang. In their amicable suggestions I refuse to recognize the assault on what is best in me. . . .
>
> They honestly may not know how much they resent my expression of self-motivation in daily life. The poison of their envy can be tucked away in attractive packages at the sight of which I am supposed to light up with delight. Some of these wrappings are good friendship, care for my health, concern for my sanity, virtue, good name. The more poisonous the content, the lovelier the wrapping is likely to be.[25]

Envy flourishes in those who refuse to take up the burden of selfhood, in those who abdicate from their own uniqueness and power of creative action, above all in those who do not truly love themselves.

> We love out of leisure from self-concern and we are always self-concerned unless we know that someone other than ourself is prepared to maintain the significance of our being.
>
> —Grace Stuart, *Narcissus*

Understood in the psychological sense, "leisure from self-concern" is surely what we mean in the life of the spirit as "the state of grace." Thus, the damaged narcissism so often produced by the mother-daughter relationship and feminine socialization can be viewed as a kind of "original sin"—few women escape its taint. To the extent that this disability produces a fear of autonomy in a young woman, it can be said to predispose her to existential despair. Whether it is the "sickness unto death" of Kierkegaard or the "madness" described by Laing and the "anti-psychiatrists," it is experienced as a dread of being, a flight from the true self. To put oneself in this condition or to knowingly will it is, in fact, to exist in a state of sin.

Women have often consoled themselves with the traditional definitions of sin, all of which are rooted in ancient notions of hubris—of actions that attempt to transcend limitation. Sin is understood as "rebellion, willful estrangement or error in performance." In the Judaeo-Christian tradition especially, sin has been equated with acts of self-assertion or pride. We tend to view sin as an extension of potency, an unwarranted act of excelling or excess. Women, in particular, are prone to this assumption, failing to recognize the roots of sin in impotence and passivity. Kierkegaard's concept of "dread" illumines another way of looking at sin:

> Thus dread is the dizziness of freedom which occurs when the spirit would posit the synthesis, and freedom then gazes down into its own possibility, grasping at finiteness to sustain itself. In this dizziness freedom succumbs. Further than this psychology cannot go and will not. That very instant everything is changed and when freedom rises again it sees that it is guilty . . .
>
> Dread is a womanish debility in which freedom swoons. Psychologically speaking, the fall into sin always occurs in impotence.[26]

Kierkegaard equates sin with the despair of "not willing to be oneself," a flight response of the individual to the dread of autonomy. Kierkegaard's cultural and historical bias is evident in his use of the term "womanish" to describe the crippled psyche, yet it may be revealing about the prevailing disposition of women. His belief in woman's natural "devotion" and "submissiveness" leads him to assume that women sin differently than men. This confusion has been a theological cliché and one more means of rationalizing the abdication of women from self-determination.[27]

For many women, sin must be equated with "a refusal to become conscious." To the dread of freedom is added the dread of guilt. The daughter, poisoned through no fault of her own, flawed and vulnerable to the distorted narcissism that afflicted her mother before her, allows herself to sink into a kind of suspended animation. She exists, self-condemned to the repetition of Life rather than its transcendence, limited in the possibilities of the self—trapped in the coffin of immanence. She has eaten poisoned fruit. What catastrophe, what apocalypse can rescue her?

The first step for any woman is the exorcism of her relationship with her own mother—dead or alive, real or mythical, loving or unloving. The second is the exorcism of her relationships with other women and the risk of reaching out to them, as well as to men, in authentic friendship. Both of these projects will demand that a woman shed the layers of feminine socialization that have poisoned these capacities; it will demand that a woman seek spiritual maturity and wholeness through androgyny.

Androgyny should be distinguished from bisexuality. Sexuality in humans is not a kind of "syzygy" (a pair, the existence of which is maintained by its essential complementarity). Rather, as endocrinological and psychological research increasingly reveal, it is a continuum. Androgyny is not a certain type of sexuality, it is the result of a dynamic interchange of energies in a continuous system. Not to progress in it would be like trying to prevent one cerebrum of the brain from interacting with the other.

Nor does androgyny mean "masculinizing" women. Rather, it means abandoning a stereotypical constellation of qualities for a dialectical sexuality, a creative selfhood. Androgyny, then, can be the link, the bridge, the turning point between heteronomy and autonomy—a step toward full personhood.

Liv Ullmann seems to describe this transition in her autobiography, *Changing:*

> I made better contact with others. I found respect when I became independent, ceased to cling. Ceased to rely so desperately on others for my own happiness.
>
> Demands and expectations on other people's behavior, in order to make me secure, vanished. Not quite. Not forever. But I never reverted to the old state . . .
>
> At times my conscience no longer bothered me because of all that I did not do and did not know. I found pleasure in my newfound ability to make my own decisions (even when they were bad), took delight in my work, in being angry, in weeping, in laughing, in living.
>
> Joy in allowing myself to be me, positive or negative.
>
> It wasn't any miracle that had changed me. I didn't live happily ever afterward. I was often afraid.

> But I was richer within; I was better friends with myself . . .
>
> I used to want to lodge in someone's pocket and be able to jump in and out whenever it suited me. Now I go around listening for cries from women who I imagine are locked in other's pockets.[28]

A woman who has unwrapped herself, who has unfurled her wholeness, who has emerged from what Kierkegaard calls "the despair of not willing to be oneself"—a woman, in short, who has come to love herself—is unafraid of loving others. Life is no longer a chess board on which men are lined up on one side, women on the other—and only opposites can touch and love and join hearts, each piece moving in rigidly defined patterns of movement, white to black, pawn to pawn. The ballet of life comes to resemble a game of chess less, Chinese checkers more.

The evolution from stereotypical female to autonomous woman does not take place at the stroke of a fairy godmother's wand. It is a slow and often painful transformation. For some it may require a lifetime. Many women who have embarked on the journey describe the initial step as the process of discerning whether they habitually behave differently with women than with men, and the decision to be oneself with both sexes. These behaviors are so compulsive at times that some women have wished they could videotape their behavior for instant replay. Those who are aware of an extreme dichotomy often need a period of "withdrawal," of intense and exclusive female companionship, until they are ready to emerge into the mainstream again. And when they do, the "re-entry" problems are often acute, not the least of which is finding men and women who are moving in the same direction. For a woman with professional clients, the change can be even more problematic, and she may have to initiate a gradual, complex process of education for her business contacts. She might have to change jobs.

Among the other signs of a change in progress are the shedding of compulsive habits of dress, hair styles and make-up, and the emergence of a personal style that enhances self-respect and individuality. Women on the road to autonomy will naturally seek out the companionship of other women experiencing a "breakthrough," and perhaps a new set of male friends. Social priorities *vis-à-vis* men and women will equalize. An evening with a female friend will be as important as one with a male friend.

Trust will be more freely given. Compliments and expressions of sincere joy at another's success will come more easily. The autonomous woman is likely to be more genuinely supportive and less sentimental in her relationships. She will enjoy greater freedom in the expression of affection with both men and women because she has the confidence of control over her own vulnerability, and is not so greedy for emotional reinforcement of her fragile ego. Her newly developed assertiveness in situations which usually elicited stock "female" responses will increase her self-confidence and genuine enjoyment of life.

Autonomous women will expect something more of their female relationships than the "huddling" that characterizes sisters from a large family, dormitory dependencies or "country club" cliques, more than the "Little Women" syndrome. There will be less empty chatter and confessional klatsches, less soap opera and shopping—more sharing and world-making enterprises.

> "Beth, Beth, you're equivocating. You're still in the closet and why? Are you still not able to love yourself, and therefore you can't really love other women? Or are you simply scared of what society can do to you if you stand up and say you love women?"
>
> "Laura, are you so sure you love yourself better than I love myself? Maybe I wish people would just stop going to bed with each other for a year! Maybe we'd all get straight in our heads then. We'd see what really connects us."
>
> —Marge Piercy, *Small Changes*

Inevitably many women will come to a point in their lives where they will experience the prospect of overwhelming fulfillment in a relationship with another woman, and the question will arise: must a total woman-to-woman relationship lead to physical intimacy?

The notion that intimate friendship must inevitably lead to sexual intimacy is a rather deterministic assumption—and surely a reflection of a narcissistic, genitalized culture. Nevertheless, sexual encounters may take place, particularly if romantic illusion intrudes—that is, the kind of love Guitton described as "the reception in oneself of an image of oneself that derives from the beloved." Friendship is precisely an attempt to transcend the projections and introjections involved in the sexual relation. Therefore, it would seem that friendship would normally exclude physical intimacies and exclusivity, for to admit them would be to alter the relationship radically.

But sexuality is a continuum, not compartmentalized and hermetically sealed off from the rest of our being. Physical, even sexual encounters do take place between women, and they should be understood in context. The fact that two close friends have never even kissed does not diminish the sexual resonance that may surround a relationship. As Lillian Hellman remarks of her friendship with "Julia":

> There were many years, almost, between that New Year's Eve and the train moving into Germany. In those years, and the years after Julia's death, I have had plenty of time to think about the love I had for her, too strong and too complicated to be defined as only the sexual yearnings of one girl for another. And yet certainly that was there. I don't know, I never cared, and it is now an aimless guessing game. It doesn't prove much that we never kissed each other; even when I leaned down in a London funeral parlor to kiss the battered face that had been so hideously put back together, it was not the awful scars that worried me: because I had never kissed her I thought perhaps she would not want it and so I touched the face instead.[29]

Kinsey (1953) and Hunt (1974) found that about one in five single women and one in ten married women eventually experience a homosexual encounter. Moreover, the intense emotionalism that often characterizes relations between women can, and often does, spill over into passion—particularly in adolescence, or in women in the process of working out an autonomous identity. To experience love for another woman, with or without sexual intimacy, should be distinguished from lesbianism, however. In the contemporary era the latter implies a commitment to a way of life, a choice of companions that automatically excludes men and an estrangement from male-dominated situations.

Throughout history lesbianism has been regarded as a sin, a crime, a mental illness, or a life-style. No single cause of homosexual preference has been satisfactorily proved, although numerous theories have been proposed. We have psychological theories: lesbianism as "emotional incest with the mother," "rejection of the mother's narrow femininity," "fear of the father, the male." We have theological theories: homosexual relations as "shameful acts against nature," "acts which lack an essential and indispensable finality," a "symbolic confusion." We have existential theories: "it is a matter of choice, arrived at in a complex total situation and based upon a free decision; no sexual fate governs the life of the individual women: her type of eroticism, on the contrary, expresses her general outlook on life." We have sociological theories: homosexual preference as "a symptom of the devaluation of the feminine in our society," or "an alternative to the indigenous masculine inadequacy and immaturity in our culture," or "a significant social protest."[30]

No one of the theories offers a total explanation of lesbianism, although all contribute something toward it. It is neither a fate, nor a perversion—it is a reality that has both personal and social roots. It is not an irreversible, determined state of being, but a preference that is forged by a series of choices in the face of circumstantial factors over a long period of time. To the extent that it is a choice, it may contribute to autonomy. (Although this effect may be obviated by the energy expended in coping with the cost of deviance, psychologically and socially.) To the extent that it is a symptom—of immaturity, of psychological deprivation, or of political alienation—it should be regarded as a transitional phase. It can be, and often is, simply another excursion into the "tyranny of the couple," an unresolved symbiotic relationship. The lesbian style of life can be simply a matter of exchanging one female-identity "formula" for another. Its cliqueishness and conformity are often evidence of this.

The current visibility of radical lesbianism, however, like the "gay" phenomenon in general, is an indication that culturally we have reached a "boundary" crisis. We have reached the absurd limits of the social tyranny of sex-role stereotyping. Sexual deviance becomes a survival mechanism in coping with the dilemma of extreme psychological polarization. In some individuals it is an acute expression of sexism (C. A. Tripp's *Homosexual Matrix* is riddled with it). In others, it is a tactic employed to cope with a condition—a political "separatism" as well as a psychological rejection of an unacceptable role.

In this respect it is significant that men often precipitate homosexual experiences before heterosexual encounters; whereas in women, they often follow years of heterosexual "normalcy." The incidence of lesbianism in separated, divorced, widowed women—as well as among prostitutes—seems to be higher than in the female population at large.

The current transsexual surgery fad is another by-product of the boundary crisis; perhaps the cruelest one. It is perhaps the most dramatic evidence of the tyranny of sex roles in our society. If sexuality was regarded as a secondary aspect of a shared humanity rather than the essence of personality, perhaps some people would find it less necessary to mutilate themselves in order to liberate their souls.

Androgyny, then, may be a necessary purge for our social malaise. As it increases, homosexuality will likely recede in social significance; instead of alternative psyches and polarized identities, life will offer many paths toward a fully developed, unique personhood—a world in which, as Anaïs Nin has suggested, the only taboo would be on not loving.

The development of androgyny, and hence the prospect of the recession of homosexuality, seems closely tied to two factors: child-rearing practices and the role of women. The experience of two cultures—China and Israel—is especially significant. The incidence of homosexuality in those cultures is apparently negligible. A psychiatrist comments on the modern Chinese approach:

> Such a system, exposing children from infancy to the care and supervision of adults other than their parents and significantly reducing the amount of time spent in the family household, does not permit the atmosphere of intense, exclusive intimacy prevailing in Western families, where all of the unconscious processes of the child's psychosexual development are focused mainly on relationships with the parents. The system therefore affords excellent protection against the development of the kinds of family patterns from which homosexuality emerges. (This interpretation is further supported by the fact that homosexuality is virtually unknown in those persons who have been raised in Israeli Kibbutzim.)
>
> The role of women in China is also extremely different from their role in the West. No Chinese woman is socialized into believing that motherhood is her primary or highest calling. Everyone is expected to work outside the home, women as well as men, and all are trained for a job or profession. Women are not excluded from any endeavor on the basis of sex alone. Clothing for men and women is, to Western eyes, similar, and in no way sexually provocative.[31]

While one might question whether a society that is free of overt deviance can be assumed to be free of it psychologically, sociological evidence suggests that homosexuality is closely tied to the patriarchal and individualistic structures that prevail in many Western cultures.

Bringing society to the point where the only taboo is on not loving, and reshaping the self to "Love and do what you will" are goals worthy of human aspiration and endeavor. Androgyny is the way to autonomy for the self and to maturity for a society. But is there more to development than autonomy?

The religious person must answer, "Yes." There is more to personal growth, there is a point of reference beyond the self that remains. The threshold of religious, theonomous existence is won only at the expense of achieving ethical autonomy. But in the encounter with the sacred order beyond the personal, we confront a finality, a design that is given. How then does our struggle to achieve androgyny—the catalyst of an autonomous existence—square with the eternal design? Is it, in fact, a contradiction of the prophetic revelations of most religions?

It would seem not, provided one sees creation as a process. If one accepts the notion of a sacred order, then human acts must be measured in the degree of their approximation to the goal of creation itself. If the sacred order prescribes (as the evolution of the cortex seems to indicate) increasing human control over the very processes of creation and over human nature itself; and if its goal is (as the evolution of higher forms seems to suggest) a cosmic convergence, then the threshold of androgyny and the liberation of women must be viewed as nothing less than a point of "critical mass" in evolution. In retrospect, the words of Galatians 3 become, not a statement of fact, not merely a symbolic cliché, but a prophecy of the coming kingdom:

> There is neither Jew nor Greek, there is neither slave nor free, there is neither male nor female, for you are all one in Christ Jesus.

Androgyny is a precondition of the liberation of a personality imprisoned in a sex role. Without it, friendship is impossible; with it, authentic sisterhood becomes a sacrament of autonomy.

Each of us has a personal Snow White script. Mine is a dream in which the dwarfs—those embryonic androgynes—are transformed into Snow White's full-grown sisters. They release her from the coffin and the poison, and together they go off to rescue the Prince!

the legend

Overtly the story helps the child to accept sibling rivalry as a rather common fact of life and promises that he need not fear being destroyed by it; on the contrary, if these siblings were not so nasty to him, he could never triumph to the same degree at the end . . . There are also obvious moral lessons: that surface appearances tell nothing about the inner worth of a person; that if one is true to oneself, one wins over those who pretend to be what they are not; and that virtue will be rewarded, evil punished.

Openly stated, but not as readily recognized, are the lessons that to develop one's personality to the fullest, one must be able to do hard work and be able to separate good from evil, as in the sorting of the lentils. Even out of lowly matter like ashes things of great value can be gained, if one knows how to do it.

—Bruno Bettelheim, *The Uses of Enchantment*[1]

The literature on female socialization reminds one of the familiar image of Cinderella's stepsisters industriously lopping off their toes and heels so as to fit into the glass slipper (key to the somewhat enigmatic heart of the prince)—when of course it was never intended for them anyway.

—Judith Long Laws, "Woman as Object"[2]

The important factor to us is Cinderella's conditioning. It is decidedly not to go on dutifully sweeping the floor and carrying the wood. She is conditioned to get the hell out of those chores. There is, the American legend tells her, a good-looking man with dough, who will put an end to the onerous tedium of making a living. If he doesn't come along (the consumer must consequently suppose), she isn't just lacking in good fortune, she is being cheated out of her true deserts. Better, says our story, go out and make the guy. In other words, we have turned the legend backwards and our Cinderella now operates as her sisters did . . .

The goal of security, seen in terms of things alone and achieved in those terms during the least secure period in human history, has predictably ruined Cinderella: she has the prince, the coach, the horses—but her soul's a pumpkin and her mind's a rat-warren. She desperately needs help.

—Philip Wylie, *Generation of Vipers*[3]

Cinderella, the best-known and probably best-liked fairy tale, is above all a success story. The rags-to-riches theme perhaps explains its equal popularity among boys as well as girls. It is a very old fairy tale, having at least 345 documented variants and numerous unrecorded versions. The iconic focus of the tale on the lost slipper and Cinderella's "perfect fit" suggests that the story may have originated in the Orient where the erotic significance of tiny feet has been a popular myth since ancient times.

The basic motifs of the story are well-known: an ill-treated heroine, who is forced to live by the hearth; the twig she plants on her mother's grave that blossoms into a magic tree; the tasks demanded of the heroine; the magic animals that help her perform the tasks and provide her costume for the ball; the meeting at the ball; the heroine's flight from the ball; the lost slipper; the shoe test; the sisters' mutilation of their feet; the discovery of the true bride and the happy marriage. The variants retain the basic motifs; while differing considerably in detail, they range more widely in their origins than any other fairy tale: Asiatic, Celtic, European, Middle-Eastern and American Indian versions numbered among them.

The Horatio Alger quality of the story helps to explain its special popularity in mercantile and capitalistic societies. As a parable of social mobility it was seized upon by the writers of the new "literature of aspiration" in the seventeenth and eighteenth centuries as a basic plot for a new kind of private fantasy—the novel. Our literary world has not been the same since *Pamela* and all her orphaned, governess sisters. Most Anglo-American novels, early and late, are written in the shadow of *Pamela* and the Cinderella myth. Even Franklin's *Autobiography,* the seminal work in the success genre, owes much to the myth. The primary "moral" of the fairy tale—that good fortune can be merited—is the very essence of the Protestant Ethic.

At the personal and psychological level, Cinderella evokes intense identification. It is a tale of sibling rivalry (and subliminally, of sex-role stereotyping)—a moral fable about socialization. Very few themes could be closer to the inner experience of the child, an emerging self enmeshed in a family network. As Bettelheim observes, it is deceptively simple in the associations it evokes:

> *Cinderella* tells about the agonies of sibling rivalry, of wishes coming true, of the humble being elevated, of true merit being recognized even when hidden under rags, of virtue rewarded and evil punished—a straightforward story. But under this overt content is concealed a welter of complex and largely unconscious material . . .[4]

The personality of the heroine is one that, above all, accepts *abasement* as a prelude to and precondition of *affiliation*. That abasement is characteristically expressed by Cinderella's servitude to menial tasks, work that diminishes her. This willing acceptance of a condition of worthlessness and her expectation of rescue (as a reward for her virtuous suffering) is a recognizable paradigm of traditional feminine socialization. Cinderella is deliberately and systematically excluded from meaningful achievements. Her stepmother assigns her to meaningless tasks; her father fails her as a helpful mentor. Her sisters, inferior in quality of soul, are preferred before her.

But Cinderella does not become a teenage runaway, nor does she wreak any kind of Gothic sabotage on the family. Like many of the Jews who went to the gas chambers in World War II, she has internalized the consciousness of the victim. She really believes she belongs where she is. The paradox of this acceptance of a condition of worthlessness in the self, along with a conviction of the ultimate worthiness and heroism of one's role, is part of the terrible appeal of the fairy tale. For women, especially, it is both mirror and model. Perrault's version of the tale ends with a pointed poetic moral:

> 'Tis that little gift called grace,
> Weaves a spell round form and face . . .
> And if you would learn the way
> How to get that gift today—

How to point the golden dart
That shall pierce the Prince's heart—
Ladies, you have but to be
Just as kind and sweet as she!

Cinderella's place by the hearth and her identification with ashes suggests several associations. At the most obvious level, her place by the chimney is an emblem of her degradation. But it is also symbolic of her affinity with the virtues of the hearth: innocence, purity, nurturance, empathy, docility. Cinderella has a vestal quality that relieves her of any obligation to struggle and strive to better her world. She must apprentice herself to this time of preparation for her "real" life with the expected One.

Like most fairy tales, *Cinderella* dramatizes the passage to maturity. Her sojourn among the ashes is a period of grieving, a transition to a new self. On the explicit level of the story, Cinderella is literally grieving for her dead mother. Grimm's version of the tale preserves the sense of process, of growth that is symbolized in the narrative. Instead of a fairy godmother—*deus ex machina*—Cinderella receives a branch of a hazel bush from her father. She plants the twig over her mother's grave and cultivates it with her prayers and tears. This is her contact with her past, her roots, her essential self. Before one can be transformed one must grieve for the lost as well as the possible selves, as yet unfulfilled—Kierkegaard's existential anguish.

The mother is also identified in several variants with helpful animals, a calf, a cow, or a goat—all milk-giving creatures. In Grimm's version the magic helpers are birds that live in the magic tree. The animals assist her in the performance of the cruel and meaningless tasks her stepmother assigns. The magic trees and helpful animals are emblems of the faith and trust that is demanded of Cinderella, the belief that something good can be gained from whatever one does. There is a subliminal value implied here, that work is seldom to be enjoyed for its own sake, but only to be endured for some greater end. It is essentially a "predestined" view of work as incapable of redemption. Service at the hearth is not intrinsically worthwhile, but acquires its value through the virtue it extracts from the heroine. Significantly, when the heroine is released from her servitude, the structure of belief—the myth—collapses. Cinderella's father destroys the pear tree and the pigeon house.

The Perrault version places great emphasis on the "Midnight" prohibition given to Cinderella. A traditional connotation would, of course, associate it with the paternal mandate of obedience, and a threat: if the heroine does not return to domesticity and docility at regular intervals she may lose her "virtue" and no longer merit her expected one. Like the old conduct manuals for ladies, the moral of the tale warns against feminine excursions as well as ambition. Too much time spent "abroad" may result in indiscreet sex or unseemly hubris, or both. "No excelling" and "no excess."

As a dynamic metaphor of the feminine condition, it illuminates the double life that many women experience: the attraction of work and achievement, perhaps "celebrity," outside the home, and the emotional pull of the relationships and security within the home. For most women diurnal life is not a seamless robe. There are sharp divisions between creative work and compulsive activity, between assertiveness and passivity, between social life and domestic drudgery, between public routines and private joys. Women are, in the contemporary world, acutely aware of the need for integration. "Midnight" strikes with a terrible insistence, a cruel regularity in their lives.

Cinderella's threefold escape from the ball (Perrault's version) is of course designed to make her more desirable to the Prince. Or is it a reflection of her own ambivalence? (In Grimm's version, she is under no prohibition, she leaves of her own accord.) Bettelheim offers two interesting interpretations:

1) She wants to be "chosen" for herself, in her natural state, rather than because of a splendid appearance wrought by magic.
2) Her withdrawals show that, in contrast to her sisters, she is not "aggressive" in her sexuality but waits patiently "to be chosen."[5]

The latter interpretation is underscored by the "perfect fit" of Cinderella's foot in the slipper, and by the sisters' frantic efforts to mutilate their own feet in order to diminish their size (symbolic of their aggressive, masculine traits). Here we see the two sides of the "formula female." On the surface, perfectly conformed to the feminine stereotype; within, massive lacerations of the spirit. The slipper is indeed the ultimate symbol of "that which is most desirable in a woman," with all of its stereotypical seductiveness and destructiveness.

The slipper, the central icon in the story, is a symbol of sexual bondage and imprisonment in a stereotype. Historically, the virulence of its significance is born out in the twisted horrors of Chinese footbinding practices. On another level, the slipper is a symbol of power—with all of its accompanying restrictions and demands for conformity. When the Prince offers Cinderella the lost slipper (originally a gift of the magic bird), he makes his kingdom hers.

We know little of Cinderella's subsequent role. In Grimm's version she is revenged by the birds which pluck out the eyes of the envious sisters. But Perrault's version celebrates Cinderella's kindness and forgiveness. Her sisters come to live in the palace and marry two worthy lords. In the Norse variant of the tale, Aslaug, the heroine, marries a Viking hero, bears several sons, and wields a good deal of power in Teutonic style. (She is the daughter of Sigurd and Brynhild.) But in most tales Cinderella disappears into the vague region known as the "happily ever after." She changes her name, no doubt, and—like so many women—is never heard of again.

There are moments when all of us can find ourselves in the Cinderella tale: as bitchy, envious, desperate sibling-peers; or victim-souls like Cinderella, passive, waiting patiently to be rescued; or nasty, domineering "stepmothers," fulfilling ourselves by means of manipulative affiliations—all of them addicted to needing approval. And then we know that for the Prince we should read "Patriarchy."

THREE

Cinderella and Women's Work

"AND what are you going to be when you grow up, little girl?" The old scenario is all too familiar. We know the expected responses: "teacher, nurse, secretary." Above all, "I want to be a mommie!" For little brother, the options are considerably broadened. He can even want to be a "garbage man" in his youthful fantasies, if he wishes. If he fails to mention that he might also want to be a "daddy" someday, it is of no consequence—his chief ambition in life should be the work of the world. From the earliest years of consciousness the little boy thinks of himself as a potential *worker*. The little girl will more likely think of work as an adjunct to something else, to a *relationship*.

Ironically, when the little girl grows into a woman and assumes the most ambitious role anticipated for her—that of mommie and homemaker—she discovers the schizoid view that society takes of her role. She is the primary "transmitter and preserver of values," but often cannot get credit in her own name. She is the chief manager and dispatcher of the home, but her work is not recognized as worthy of a salary or social security benefits. She is usually the exclusive care-giver and instructor of children, but this kind of work ranks in the lowest category of skills in job classifications.

Moreover, women face two major obstacles to developing an identity as worker, maker, producer. One is the mythologizing of the mother/homemaker role, and at the same time, its devaluation in the "real" world. The other is the failure of women to see work as a necessary component of identity and autonomy. Indeed, for many women marriage and anticipated motherhood represents a release from a prison sentence: a life shackled to a nine-to-five clerical job, a role characterized by monotony, powerlessness and depersonalization. The role of mother/homemaker, by contrast, at least provides intimacy and a sense of personal power. Being queen of a small kingdom is better than being a lackey in a large one—or so it may seem, for a time.

Later, the uneasiness will set in. The panic and the rage. The monotony, the trivialization of energy, the social isolation can overwhelm the housewife. If she escapes a major breakdown, she may find herself in mid-life struggling with a new scenario. If she lived out the expected answer to the old question, "And what do you want to be when you grow up, little girl?"—she may suddenly be asking herself, "What do I want to be when my children grow up?" The world, in fact, may seem for time about ready to swallow her up. These apocalyptic feelings in her maturity are the tragic result of exclusion from work that might have given her a sense of control over her world, her destiny, and her soul.

> The overt hustling society is the microcosm of the rest of the society. The power relationships are the same and the games are the same. Only this one I was in control of. The greater one I wasn't. In the outside society, if I tried to be me, I wasn't in control of anything. As a bright, assertive woman, I had no power. As a cold, manipulative hustler, I had a lot. I knew I was playing a role. Most women are taught to *become* what they act. All I did was act out the reality of American womanhood.
>
> —Roberta Victor, Hooker, quoted in Studs Terkel, *Working*

One of the great paradoxes about the progress of developing societies is that it is often achieved at the expense of a regression in women's function and status. While it is true that in most societies—primitive, ancient and modern—some division between male and female roles has prevailed, industrialization has exaggerated and radicalized these divisions. Primitive and even colonial women played a much more integral role in the business of survival. Their identity as workers and managers was taken for granted. The "valiant woman" described in Proverbs 31 is high in self-esteem and in the eyes of the community because her role is integral to the private and public life of the community.

In our own culture women of the colonial and frontier eras were closely tied to the economic enterprises of the emerging society.[6] The housewife supervised perhaps a score of trades that were vital to the subsistence of the emerging settlements and villages. During the seventeenth century, when spinning and weaving were household industries performed primarily by women and children, each household provided its own raw materials and produced chiefly to meet its own needs. But it was not uncommon for women to market part of their output. Later merchants contracted with women to spin yarn in their own homes. The first factories were simply depots for gathering work which had been contracted to local households. The colonial woman functioned not only as the foreman of this embryonic factory, but also as a superintendent of welfare services. Town officers and justices of the peace often sent widows, orphans, the poor and even criminals into respectable homes for care and rehabilitation. While the letter of the law permitted women a modicum of legal authority and autonomy, nevertheless colonial court records indicate that they occasionally asserted their economic importance by bringing suit and often by inserting "rights" clauses in colonial deeds and other transactions. In effect, women of the colonial era were not forced to choose between work and domesticity as alternative vocations. Domestic work was, in fact, often performed by unmarried young women in order to free the married woman for work in the family industry. Ironically, the work roles of married and unmarried women have been reversed in modern times.

Thus, industrialization brought a divergence, a dichotomy. The division between the world of work and the home became acute. What began as a condition of efficiency and hyper-production ended as a social stratification: a split between a *servant* caste and a caste of *autonomous* individuals along sexual lines. Men, who would busy themselves in the work of the world, would be *autonomous*. Women, who would anchor and "manage" the home, would be *supportive,* dependent—their engagement with the world vicarious.

However, to explain the contemporary situation of women, something more than a change in the locus of productive work must be acknowledged. Woman's attitude toward work changed radically. How and when did this happen? Again, one must look to the effects of industrialization, particularly to the early Republican era in America.

By mid-eighteenth century, land grants had been depleted and the old town practice of distributing fields and meadows gratis was discontinued. Land along the Eastern seaboard now became prey to private enterprise, to be won or lost according to one's relative purchasing power. Money and mobility displaced subsistence and stability as the American economy began to shift from an agrarian to an industrial base. Small farming communities were transformed into stratified societies, where the top 10 per cent of the population often controlled more than half of the total wealth. Thus, the advent of a commercial economy heralded new divisions between neighbors as well as between husbands and wives.

The dissociation of home and work disrupted the integral relationship of women with the commonwealth and isolated her in a privatized sphere of domestic responsibility. As a few wealthy families came to monopolize the commerce of the eighteenth century, the primary role of the wives and daughters of the new merchant class changed from an instrumental to an expressive mode. Social mobility reduced the female role to an ornamental and utilitarian one, in the sense that the woman was expected to consolidate the family fortune through a well-calculated marriage and to reflect the status of her family by conspicuous personal adornment and social graces.

A plethora of advice-mongers in the post-Revolutionary era cautioned women against qualities of assertiveness and resourcefulness (once characteristic of their grandmothers, but now regarded as exclusively masculine traits) and admonished them to leave the "world of affairs" to men and turn their attention solely to the art of polishing husbands' and children's manners, and, of course, the silverware. Trivial duties became weighted with profound significance.

Moreover, piety, delicacy, gentility (in contrast to the rugged virtues) had now become an index of social mobility, and women were the chief emblems of success. The ethos of capitalism viewed the "leisured woman"—the woman emancipated from work—as the first fruits of "progress."

> For the middle-class woman, the doctrine of feminine domesticity was well-established by the mid-nineteenth century: marriage had become a fulltime occupation. It was, moreover, an oc-

> cupation in which women could play the role of "leisured lady!" Though evident among the aristocracy in the eighteenth century, the idle dependence of the married woman became a practicable ideal for the rising middle classes with industrialization. The idleness of a man's female dependents at home became a mark of prosperity for the Victorian middle-class role: The successful business man delighted to show off his wife and daughters expensively clad, living a life of ease and elegance.[7]

The Victorian cult of "true womanhood" denigrated work as a dimension of virtue and a moral necessity. The myth of the leisured lady endowed the middle-class woman with more protection, more pedestal-worship, and more restriction. The more idealized her role, the narrower it became. By implication, it denigrated the role of the working-class woman, driven by necessity to work—degraded in the eyes of her more affluent sisters and by the dehumanized labor that was her only option. Thus, work itself came to be seen as an unfortunate social condition, a "fall from grace." The practice of female idleness spread through the middle class until work for women became "a misfortune and a disgrace." In time, the prospect of women leaving the home for work inevitably came to be regarded as a kind of "mortal sin" against the family.

Perhaps the most important contribution of the socialistic and utopian communities that flourished in America in the nineteenth century was the riposte that they represented to this prevailing ethos. At a time when the labor of men was spiritualized and romanticized (to varnish its oppressive aspects) and when women's release from work was regarded as a kind of seal of redemption, most of the communal societies proposed social structures in which work was shared equally, inside and outside the home, and in which duties were not dichotomized along sexual lines. If human nature at times regressed to conventional and traditional behavior, at least these societies conceived of alternative modes of arranging the social contract around a more egalitarian concept of work. The practical experiments of the twentieth century were to prove more successful.

Work is, in fact, the prerequisite for acceptance in many contemporary societies: the Soviet, China, Israel. Women are not exempted from this obligation, nor is release from it seen as a kind of reward for achievement. In these societies, a woman would have to explain why she is not working. In America, she has to explain why she is working.[8] While in many of these countries the tyranny of sex-linked occupations has not been overcome, nevertheless women do not labor invisibly as they do in our culture, where work is regarded as an adjunct activity—yet where 42 per cent of the work force is female. In a society like ours, where the GNP and profit are the ultimate criteria, where economic gain is the prime rationale for behavior, the concept of satisfying work as an essential component of personal growth and collective equilibrium is generally ignored. Work is more often regarded as a means, not an end, in the American scheme of things. This attitude underlies a good deal of the rationalizing of women's exclusion from significant work roles. Why should women want to join the rat race? Men are really worse off. And so the myths multiply. As long as we continue to espouse a utilitarian view of work, there is little chance that American women will break out of the clerical/maintenance caste in which they are now imprisoned. The alienating aspects of work in a post-industrial era are undoubtedly a deterrent, but they are not an argument for allowing one half of the population to avoid responsibility for that work. Rather, the debilitating aspects of contemporary work are a challenge, a summons to deepen involvement and commitment—on the part of women as well as men—to the work of reorganizing, repatterning the structures of work.

. . . I can't find any occupation for myself. He is lucky to be so clever and talented. But I'm neither the one nor the other. One can't live on love alone . . .

It isn't hard to find work, but before doing anything one has to create some enthusiasm for breeding hens, tinkling the piano, and reading a lot of silly books and a few very good ones, or pickling cucumbers and what not . . .

If I am no good to him, if I am merely a doll, a *wife*, and not a *human being*—then it is all useless and I don't want to carry on this existence. Of course I am idle, but I am not idle by nature; I simply haven't yet discovered what I can do here . . .

I love nothing and no one except Lyova. And yet one ought to have something else to love as well, just as Lyova loves his *work* . . .

My existence is so deadly dull, while his is so full and rich, with his work and genius and immortal fame . . .

> It is sad that my emotional dependence on the man I love should have killed so much of my energy and ability; there was certainly once a great deal of energy in me.
>
> —Sophie Tolstoy, Wife, quoted in *Revelations, Diaries of Women*

If the cultural milieu has circumscribed woman in a narrow sphere of expectations and limited her aspirations to creative work, her socialization has limited her psychologically. What history has accomplished from without, socialization has accomplished within.

Women, more than men, tend to assume that the most important choice in life—or what they assume will be the most important choice—should come first in point of time. That is, the choice of a relationship. Men are more likely to give themselves first to a project—to the choice of work. Although a relationship may intervene, they seem instinctively to assume that work is the primary and initial means to identity. Women bypass or postpone this apprenticeship, to their great detriment. Many women regard their "working" time before marriage as a waiting period—a kind of limbo before one's "real" life begins, the life of relationship. A life best described by Veblen in *Theory of the Leisure Class* as "the vicarious life."

In treating this period of life as a temporary and less desirable state, in refusing to take work seriously as a personal project, women deprive themselves of one of the most essential components of identity and personhood, and one of the most essential components of a mature and lasting relationship. Work—consciously chosen, and creatively structured—is a "soul-making" process which results in a personality that not only has more to give, but needs the other person less compulsively. Simone de Beauvoir has described the connection between work and the capacity for growth, for transcendence, that is so often absent in women because of their own acquiescence or inertia. The husband goes beyond the confines of the family to a productive role in society. He experiments with new selves in assuming new, challenging tasks. He expands his own future by cooperating in the construction of the collective future. "He incarnates transcendence." The woman at home is chained to the continuation of the species and to the maintenance of the family unit. She is rooted in immanence.

The tension between these two functions of maintenance and

progression finds a happy synthesis in the husband's experience. His occupation and public presence give him a personal sense of change, growth and progression. When the need for security and reassurance, for sameness, overtakes him, he has a home to retreat to. Although it is a necessary anchorage, it never becomes an end in itself. The woman, however, deprived of a complementary experience, struggles to set up "a universe of permanence and continuity." Her work not only gives her no autonomy, it dooms her to disappointment. Even for her children, life exists beyond the family limits. A woman's work takes on dignity and meaning only when it is linked to significant "others" who are able to transcend themselves in productive involvement in society.[9]

De Beauvoir unequivocally proposes the entry of women in to male-dominated spheres and the adoption of "male" economic roles by females. She is concerned about the liberation of women but somewhat unconcerned about the liberation of work. (Significantly, the second half of her book, *The Second Sex,* although it is the primer of the women's movement, is arranged more or less in a sequence that reflects women's relationships—"The Married Woman," "The Mother," "The Woman in Love," etc.—with nary a chapter devoted to the qualitative and psychological aspects of the work of the world.) The denigration of work associated with the home is the corollary of uncritical acceptance of the preferred status of patriarchal work patterns. De Beauvoir's uncritical treatment of the masculine sphere and simplistic view of the feminine sphere does not negate her argument, but does leave the task of liberation somewhat incomplete.

Without work, however, the road to transcendence—to autonomy—is blocked. Full development of personality implies growth, a succession of acts of self-transcendence. Or as the philosophers put it, "selfhood consists in a continual relationship to the possible."

The truth is, that women who discover fulfillment through work and professional effort find the same satisfaction as men. When performed with discipline, integrity and fidelity, it produces recognizable virtues—detachment from ego, self-pity and arrogance. Glenda Jackson, whose self-image is that of an "artist" rather than a "star," sums it up: "What is important is the work you are doing, now how you feel." The comment illuminates the difference between the joy of accomplishment that some realize and the mere sentimental dedication that many women experience.

Many women would, in fact, find this kind of fulfillment difficult to imagine if it implied singleness or childlessness. A recent study reveals that many of these fears are based on myth rather than reality.[10] The study, conducted by Kathryn Welds of the Payne Whitney Psychiatric Clinic of New York Hospital, was designed to test both the popular view of the voluntarily childless as "unhappy, selfish, lonely, immature, and emotionally unstable," and a developmental theory of one of the leading psychoanalytic thinkers of our time, Erik Erikson. Erikson held that to avoid psychological stagnation, most human beings must undertake the task of bearing and rearing the next generation in order to reach full maturity. The findings of the study indicate, on the contrary, that the ego maturity associated with adulthood—"generativity"—can be achieved by those who are not biologically generative or are not engaged in specifically nurturant roles. Moreover, high levels of occupational productivity and job satisfaction seemed to correlate with low levels of anxiety and a high index of maturity. Thus, one of the most serious obstacles to feminine fulfillment in work—the assumption that postponing children, or the election of childlessness may retard one's own psychological development—is one more myth that must be overcome.

Indications are that work, a fulfilling career or commitment to a project of some sort, is in fact the best preparation for motherhood. A high degree of interest and involvement in some kind of work is often the best prognosis for enjoyment of and success in the role of motherhood. As Sidney Callahan observes, "A strong, active, secure mother with her own goals can be the mother who gives security to her child and activates his goal-directed behavior. A good worker or good mother has the wherewithal to raise good children." Some women combine both roles successfully:

> They have the pleasures of working and the joys of motherhood. Many of these women find that combining work and motherhood makes them better at both. Work takes up their aggressive energies to shape and achieve, and keeps their children from being unduly worked on. They can relax with their children and relate to them as persons rather than as projects or jobs. Their mutual dialogue with their children is enhanced by their work outside of the domestic sphere.[11]

Choosing a work that is financially rewarding as well as personally gratifying may be a precondition of fulfillment in the paramount relationships of life. Young women should be encouraged to make this choice first, instead of belatedly, often in the midst of a mid-life crisis. A woman who is able to support herself in work she enjoys gains an irreplaceable sense of competence—the kind of competence that is essential for self-validation and social identity. If women are excluded from "cooperative participation in the technologies of a culture" and from "the completion of tasks," they are dwarfed spiritually as well as socially. If women are unskilled and inexperienced in work, in the shaping of environment, they cannot be free from economic dependency (and hence, emotional dependency) on someone else.

Women, in short, must be trained, coaxed or dragged—kicking and screaming, if necessary—out of their "socially sanctioned existential cowardice." Work is crucial in this transformation.

> We do not exist in order to work, but we work in order to be.
>
> —Rosemary Ruether, Theologian, quoted in *Women: New Dimensions*

Recovery of the spiritual sense of work is imperative if women are to be liberated rather than automated by it. The idea of work as "a command to self-transcendence" is rooted in the Judaeo-Christian heritage. Greco-Roman, biblical and medieval sources alike confirm this consciousness. It is one of the distinguishing characteristics of Western civilization as a whole. As an ethical principle it reached a kind of apotheosis in Protestant theology with the doctrine of a "calling." In our own culture, attitudes toward work as well as our entire economic system are rooted in religious concepts which underlie the idea of a calling; self-scrutiny and asceticism, stewardship of goods, democratic covenant and the coming kingdom. In its inception, the capitalistic ethos celebrates the spiritual sense of work. Unfortunately, its very success in time diminished its moral and spiritual motive—industrialization resulted in production for the sake of unlimited profits, in alienation of workers from their products, and in the establishment of artificial hierarchies of activity. The ancient parable of Cain and Abel has been re-enacted many times in history.

Slavery came into existence among the Greeks when they began to denigrate certain kinds of human labor. Women were relegated to an inferior caste probably as early as the iron age, and most dramatically with the coming of industrialization. "Woman's work" was segregated from significant human activity.

Recovery of the spiritual sense of work and the moral imperative it contains demands that women not abdicate—as men once did—from the nurturant, hearth-centered labor that they have known, but that this be integrated with the achieving, world-shaping enterprises they have generally avoided. Likewise, their liberation can be fulfilled only if men integrate their one-sided, competitive, worldly pursuits with the private sphere of home maintenance and child rearing. Women will never be equal on the job until the economic relations of the family and employment are restructured in concert. As long as working women have to solve the problem of the double shift—home and work—only the unmarried or childless are likely to maintain significant careers. Those who are heads of households are forced into desperate compromises which may leave the home neglected. Women are made to feel guilty for this situation, instead of society assuming responsibility for inventing new solutions to the problem.

There are no models in our civilization to inspire this change. It will perhaps be more difficult for men than for women. Ultimately, we must evolve an ecological model of work—one that sees all functions as equally important in sustaining an equilibrium in society as well as in the personality. Feminist theologian Sheila Collins described these interrelationships and systematic interconnections between patriarchal structures, work patterns and sexual roles:

> Racism, sexism, class exploitation, and ecological destruction are four interlocking pillars upon which the structure of the patriarchy rests. The structures of oppression are everywhere the same, although the particular forms in which oppression is manifested may at first glance look different. The democracy of the Athenian polis, to which the Western world has always looked as its ideal, was made possible only through the restricted domestic labors of the slaves and wives of the Athenian property owners. Western "freedom" and affluence depend on the domestication of women and the exploitation of a low-paid labor base made up of minorities and women as well as unlimited access to

> foreign sources of natural resources which are taken from the ground without regard for the rights of the earth or the people who live on the land.
>
> The feminist experience has thus enabled us to penetrate the superficial differences to see the systemic and psychic links between the various forms of injustice. Feminists hold that the alienation of woman from man—because it was the first and still is the longest lasting form of human alienation—can be seen as a primordial paradigm from which all other unjust relationships derive.[12]

Across the synapses of history, humanity is shaping itself into a microcosm of earth, of the cosmos. To resist this convergence, this integration within the individual personality, is as futile and sterile as it would be for an entire culture to consciously resist change. Old boundaries and dichotomies are blurring. Primitive divisions of role, hierarchies of activity, pyramids of value are collapsing in the emergence of this new world view. Women are intimately catalytic in this change. Work is at the very core of this emerging ecosystem.

Those who have accepted the Genesis prescription as the norm for human labor—"thou shalt earn thy bread by the sweat of thy brow"—are in need of the good news. The message of the Gospel is perhaps best expressed in Romans 8: "For the creation waits with eager longing for the revelation of the sons of God; for the creation was subjected to futility, not of its own will but by the will of him who subjected it in hope; because the creation itself will be set free from its bondage to decay and obtain the glorious liberty of the children of God." The liberation theologians have recalled humanity to the spiritual dimension of work. To work, to transform this world, is to become a person and to build the human community; it is also to save. Building the temporal city is not simply a stage of humanization; it is in itself the redemption that embraces the entire cosmos.

Teilhard de Chardin, in 1927, anticipated much of the world view emerging today when he observed that "fidelity" required more than obedience and docility to Christian/human values. One must also "construct"—starting from the most natural zone of his own self—a work, an opus, into which something enters from all the elements of the earth. "One makes his own soul" and at the same time collaborates in another work, the completion of the world. In describing the way in which work overcomes existential inertia,

Teilhard observes that those who work learn to abandon over and over again the form that their labor or art first takes. Those who work honestly and creatively learn detachment, asceticism and the transcendence of self.[13]

The passivity and privatization of women in our society are the most serious obstacles to their own autonomy and personal growth, and also to the transformation and redemption of the entire social structure. Women, on the whole, are not convinced that they are needed in, or need activity in, the public sphere. This attitude has made it easier for society to create a false and artificial dichotomy between the public and private sphere, with all of the double standards, dualisms and one-sidedness (neuroses) that this implies. Likewise, men have not been convinced that they are needed in, or should participate in, the hearth-centered private sphere.

Thus, in the hierarchy of motives for work, women do not often aspire to goals beyond the most elementary. A scheme of motives might be arranged as follows, moving from the minimally to maximally transcendent:

1. subsistence, survival
2. human dignity, security
3. "sense of duty"—social approval
4. increased status, "the good life"
5. pleasure, significance—creative fulfillment
6. redemption of the social order, "the future"

Few women aspire to or find it possible to work at the higher levels of transcendence. Most women work because they have to, or feel they must, or as a diversion from their primary social role. Hence, the "job" is inevitably an activity that is alienated from being. With rare exceptions, work outside the home seldom grows organically out of the roots of a woman's identity. It is not part of her, and thus it is often joyless and mechanized. It is chosen not for itself, but for ultimately utilitarian motives.

The argument that women's exclusion from a broad range of skills and competencies by reason of social attitudes and/or discrimination is the chief obstacle to be overcome is a fallacy. The first obstacle is not lack of skills, but passivity—a mind-set that would prefer to react rather than initiate, to nurture rather than construct, to support rather than command, to tidy up the universe rather than disturb it.

In his fascinating history of working men and women, called *Working,* Studs Terkel found a few exceptions to the rather bleak aspect that women's work presents on the whole. Kay Stepkin is a twenty-nine-year-old woman who has taken a minimal skill, a hearth-centered activity—breadmaking—and transformed it into a revolutionary and transcendent form of work—a Bakery Cooperative that has helped to reshape a neighborhood. The "organic" origins of her idea are evident:

> It was about nine years ago. I would read books on it. But there was no one to talk to. I was doing different jobs. I was teaching. I was a waitress. I never did anything satisfying. About two years ago, I started realizing how bad things really are out here—on the planet . . .
>
> I see us living in a completely schizophrenic society. We live in one place, work in another place, and play in a third. You have to talk differently depending on who you're talking to. You work in one place, get to know the people, you go home at night and you're lonely because you don't know anyone in your neighborhood. I see this as a means of bringing all that together.[14]

There is a consciousness in Kay that her work is self-fulfilling and self-transcending, and there is also an overwhelming sense of "gift"—a work that transcends and liberates the social order. The Bakery Cooperative deliberately contradicts the hierarchical, patriarchal structure of most American businesses. Authority is participatory: "We have men and women, we all do the same kind of work. Everyone does everything . . . Different people take responsibility for different jobs . . . Everything we do is completely open. We do the baking right out here. People in the neighborhood, waiting for the bus in the morning, come in and watch us make bread." Harmony with the ecological system is a priority: "We don't like to waste anything. That's real important. We use such good ingredients, we hate to see it go into a garbage can. And it may be burned and go into the air some way . . . Were looking for ways to get our product to people cheaper without resorting to machinery." The cooperative reunites the worker and the product by eliminating middlemen, exploitative profit and unnecessary overhead. They grind their own grain. Customers bring their own bags.

Most of all, the experiences of the Bakery Cooperative, a unique amalgam of hearth-centered function and public business, has restored a sense of joy in work for its own sake.

> Work is an essential part of being alive. Your work is your identity. It tells you who you are. It's gotten so abstract. People don't work for the sake of working. They're working for a car, a new house, or a vacation. It's not the work itself that's important to them. There's such a joy in doing work well.[15]

Kay's evaluation of her work experience reveals some of the elements that make work pleasurable for its own sake: the sense of being needed, interaction with peers, problem solving and decision making, a sense of novelty and excitement, having impact on the surrounding milieu, a pride in craft and product. The more these elements are present in the work experience, the more transcendent it becomes. All too often, the American housewife enjoys only the pleasure of being needed, and when she is no longer needed there are no other joys to evoke satisfaction. The "empty nest" and the widowed years can be devastating for women who have never learned the value of work for its own sake, who have never explored alternative selves in various work roles.

For many women, the problem with work is the same as the problem with orgasm. They can't enjoy it because they can't enjoy themselves. The psychological blocks to ecstasy and pleasure have to be removed; the sense of inferiority, the need for approval, the dependency on a "relationship" for all fulfillment. Most women live life in the imperative mode, convinced that "I must do this" rather than "I want to do this," or "I enjoy doing this, therefore I will do it." One cannot lose oneself in a work unless one has at least a modicum of identity and autonomy; yet it seems that one cannot acquire identity and autonomy without some participation in the world of work.

The denigration of "women's work" has contributed to a mindset that denies the value of certain kinds of work and therefore inhibits pleasure in it. Homemaking, child rearing, secretarial work—although sex-linked and often restrictive occupations—nevertheless have their own intrinsic pleasures. Zen can be invoked to exorcise and transcendentalize everything from corporate decision making to motorcycle maintenance because these work roles are culturally valued, linked as they are to the masculine ambience of the dominant cultural ethos. We have yet to see a best seller entitled *Zen and the Art of Garbage Disposal,* or *Inner Cooking.* Perhaps when enough men opt to share the hearth-centered functions with women, we will see an increase in this kind of treatise. Or, if enough women and men begin to share the public and private dimensions of work and fuse them in an individualized, organic rhythm, perhaps we will no longer need to invoke Zen to exorcise the ennui of stereotyped work roles.

But not everyone is free enough of the "system" to evolve an organic work life. Some jobs simply cannot be transcendentalized. Many women are trapped in these "no exit," "no escalator" situations. Another of Studs Terkel's interviewees, Nora Watson, an editor in a large publishing firm, describes the predicament:

> Jobs are not big enough for people. It's not just the assembly line worker whose job is too small for his spirit, you know? A job like mine, if you really put your spirit into it, you would sabotage immediately. You don't care. So you absent your spirit from it. My mind has been so divorced from my job, except as a source of income, it's really absurd . . .
>
> You invest a job with a lot of values that the society doesn't allow you to put into a job. You find yourself like a pacemaker that's gone crazy or something.

But to change the pacemaker would require anesthetizing the entire socioeconomic system. Impossible. The answer, for many women, seems to lie in some sort of separate peace that one must seek and make with her own situation, some psychic equilibrium that can be achieved within the scope of her indentured status. For someone like Nora Watson it means:

> You recognize yourself as a marginal person. As a person who can give only minimal assent to anything that is going on in this society . . . What you have to find is your own niche that will allow you to keep feeding and clothing and sheltering yourself without getting downtown. (Laughs) Because that's death. That's really where death is.[16]

Marginality is to be preferred to narcotization, to be sure. Although it is a tragic admission of failure, it may become an instrument of change. Flexible working hours and a shorter work week are accidental by-products of increasing marginality of workers. Women, especially, are pressing for retention of full-time status with a condensed work week (salaries pro-rated, benefits retained). They have been successful in several corporations. The arrangement (a four-day work week) gives them the freedom to seek more meaningful work (generally unpaid) on their "off" days, care for their families, etc. Then when their weekly "midnight" strikes, they change back into corporate "pumpkins." Cinderella reversed. If work and life cannot be integrated, they can at least be given equal time.

> One exciting thing for me has been the evolution of the mind. I wasn't as sharp intellectually when I was in my twenties. Oh, I got good grades and all that sort of thing. But my mind wasn't as sharp in creative thought. Research forces one to become creative and quick. And contrary to physical abilities, which unfortunately decline after the twenties, the mental capabilities seem to improve with age!
>
> My mind has become a good friend! I know I'll never be bored. I'm not afraid of the unknown because I know I can go out and do whatever I want to do.
>
> —Patricia Ann Straat, Biochemist, Space Biologist, quoted in *Conversations: Working Women Talk About Doing a Man's Job*

Early feminists were fond of citing "penis-deprivation"—in all of its symbolic connotations—as the chief obstacle to women's upward mobility in professional work roles. Today, it is more likely to be their failure to manipulate other appendages—slide rules, computers, calculators—that holds women back. More crucially, their failure to master the special languages and dialects of numbers, of finance, of technology reduces them to "immigrant" status in many male-identified fields. Inevitably, many women are trapped in the job ghetto. Having been put through the double strainer of socialization and education, occupational segregation will finally enclose their aspirations within permanent boundaries.

The "tracking" that will shape a woman's work trajectory begins early; as early as her first dollhouse and tea set (when she might have preferred, or should have been given, an erector set!); as early as her first interest in cosmetics (when everyone assumes that she has no curiosity about mechanics); as early as her unsuccessful attempts to be a paper boy or play on the block football team. The tyranny of the "formula"—the requirements for "femininity," for making it as a woman—sets up a deterrence pattern. "Math anxiety" will overtake most girls while they are still in elementary school, and by the time they are adolescents many will be underachievers, carefully rationing their responses in high school physics classes so as not to "scare off" the boys. Worse yet, many will simply drift into curriculum tracks that dead-end in the job ghetto, never knowing what options they might have achieved in more substantive courses. If by some chance they do emerge from high school with high College Board scores in math and ambitions for theoretical physics or high finance, college will considerably dampen their enthusiasm, particularly the experience of quality "coeducational" universities, where many pre-professional programs continue to be "male preserves." Women, by this time, track themselves out of these areas because of social anxieties, subtle harassments, cutthroat competition—and frequently, out of boredom and exasperation with the mechanistic teaching styles that prevail in many of these fields.

For every woman who breaks precedent by entering a male-identified field, a dozen others will withdraw or de-escalate their advance, only to swell the tide of women flowing into traditional work roles—often because in mastering male-identified competencies they did not automatically acquire the confidence or determination necessary to sustain a career in these fields. Emotional rather that cognitive hurdles slow their progress and diminish their persistence. Women, in general, experience an emotional alienation from technology that continually undermines their ability to perform. Here again, a woman is victimized in a double sense. Convinced that she is inadequately equipped for higher cognitive skills and seduced into more personalized intellectual and vocational pursuits, nevertheless she is persuaded that the technology she has had no role in developing will ultimately save her. Whether it is the pill, the can opener or the dishwasher, the development of household appliances has, in fact, reduced women to a servant caste whose greatest skill is consumerism. Studies indicate that housewives are more immured in the household in direct proportion to the increase in so-called labor-saving devices. "Dependent upon technology, but removed from its sources and, paradoxically, enslaved by it, women may well have developed deep-seated resentments that persist even in those who consider themselves liberated."[17]

If contemporary females exhibit an aversion for professions like engineering, nevertheless they are flocking into law, business, and media-related fields. Samuel Florman's recent hypothesis that women are too elitist to enjoy engineering, or that they are too bemused by the seductions of "power" to pursue craft-oriented vocations, seems rather hyperbolic. The fact is, women are flocking into the professions of opinion and of personal relations because that is where they feel most comfortable and competent. Professions that are verbally oriented are naturals for women who have learned their lessons as little girls all too well. Theoretical abstractions and the intricacies of technology were off-limits for most young female minds —can we expect them to suddenly reverse their orientation at the point of career choice?

But the challenge is there. Many young women can and should make the leap. More importantly, parents and educators have to reshape the early years of female socialization which produce a perception of such limited options at the point of maturity.

Many women are finding it imperative to attempt to recover those "lost" capacities, curiosities, fascinations that they experienced as children, but which were inevitably plowed under in their subsequent cultivation as females. Women are taking courses in auto mechanics and hydraulics, in architecture and astronomy, in agriculture and law enforcement—recouping in mid-life the experimental space that life denied them in youth. For many women re-entry into the academic and vocational system in their middle years is a necessity if they are to overcome spiritual inertia and recover the roots of their identity. They should respect this need to reclaim their authentic being and not smog it over with the mere pursuit of "credentials," although that may indeed be an important element in the total process. Fidelity to the special energies that life endowed us with initially, the reintegration of a "usable past" with the possible "here and now" is absolutely essential.

For other women it will be necessary to break with the past, to test and experiment with new styles of life, to explore new modes of creativity and generativity outside conventional structures. To dwell constantly on "what might have been," to dream of a magic rescue into liberated autonomy without experiencing a gradual, patient and ascetic growth process is a futile, illusory and, at worst, neurotic expectation. Cinderella must befriend what is natural and authentic in her deepest self—symbolized by the birds and the hazel tree—leave behind what is artificial or atrophying, and then she must cease waiting, cease being in the words of Grimm, "a little stunted kitchen-wench."

But what to do? Cinderella has been brainwashed into a "supportive" mind-set, persuaded that the chief end of work is service rather than work for its own sake. At the normal transition points in her life, whether it is graduation from high school or college, or the threshold of the empty nest or widowhood, a woman has few options. Wherever she works, whatever she does, she is likely to become part of a support system for the promotion and preservation of male power. Even as a junior scientist at NASA or an executive trainee at IBM, her role will mimic—in perhaps more subtle ways—the role played by the masses of working women in secretarial and clerical jobs.

Business courses, secretarial manuals and training programs reinforce a woman's socialization as "care giver" rather than initiator, manager or policy maker. Gradually, women are prepared for and initiated into a work ghetto, "the last plantation."* Women are not only channeled into female-identified work roles through job segregation, they are also ghettoized in those roles. A recent study revealed that women tend to be concentrated in particular areas of the office or factory, and that they usually receive the same proportion of office space as they do of pay—20 per cent to 50 per cent less than what men doing roughly the same work in the same office receive.[18] Low pay and minimal benefits, dead-end jobs, sexual harassment, "efficiency" quotas, paternalism, condescension, hostility—why do women put up with it?

As Phyllis Chesler points out,

> A woman doesn't decide that she would rather make $5,000 [*sic*] a year as a nurse than a quarter of a million as a physician. Women don't decide they would rather be housewives, with no income, or recipients of welfare, than be economically independent. No one is born believing that her destiny is to await being overtaken by the "maternal instinct." Yet, it isn't necessarily because of economic philosophy that women have remained outside the American capitalist mainstream. As a matter of fact, women have been very much a part of "the system," but as its victims, and not as its beneficiaries.[19]

Women generally have had only horizontal options in a selective territory staked out for "women's work." But the deterministic argu-

* Women are concentrated chiefly into twenty of the 480 job categories listed by the Labor Department, most of them *clerical*, such as secretarial or bookkeeping, or *service*, such as sales clerks, nurses aides and waitresses.

ment does not explain the massive inertia that seems to characterize women caught in these roles. Too often, Cinderella believes that she belongs where she is. The subtle argument of the service ethic is heard most often in her own mind. For many women, "real life" remains at home. Work is something to be gotten through, to be endured until one can return to the real job—homemaking. Although these women may work outside the home all their lives, they never accept their work as a necessary and fundamental aspect of their human contribution. It is not significant or real; it is only a form of auxiliary maintenance.

Some women are seduced by another myth, the myth of the "happy work family." Middle-aged women are especially vulnerable to the gratitude trap—"I'm so grateful I could find this job, I wouldn't dare ask for what I deserve." The scenario is familiar; one woman describes a typical situation in these terms:

> Most of the people who work here are in their forties. The college would rather hire somebody in their forties or fifties. If they haven't had jobs before, or if they don't want to go too far from home, they're only too happy to get a job [here], only too willing to take less pay. It's good for [the college] because employees won't be so dissatisfied with their jobs and they'll plug along. They want you to feel [the college] is very maternal. It's a suffocating type of feeling. There's a sickening-sweet atmosphere.[20]

The "Girl Friday" myth is a far more insidious variation of the service ethic. A secretary (the kind that most men want) is a kind of wife—her job in the corporate office mimics and parodies the role of the wife in the family structure.[21] If the wife at home packs her husband's suitcase, the secretary makes his plane reservations; if the wife protects him from the children, the secretary guards him from subordinates; if the wife pays the household bills, the secretary does his expense account; if the wife listens to his office problems, the secretary is the confidant of his domestic problems; if the wife manages his social schedule, the secretary organizes and "prioritizes" his business life. A secretary (sometimes she is an "assistant" this or that) makes it possible for many men to abdicate even from responsibility for the personal dimension in their own lives; it is she who functions as his "personal" memory, remembering birthdays, anniversaries, watering his plants, handling liaisons, writing personal letters, reminding him to take his pills, call his mother. To the extent that the

Girl Friday absorbs these personal as well as menial tasks, she participates in a conspiracy (albeit unconscious) to sustain the caste system that characterizes work in "developed" societies, the division between a servant-support caste (made up of women and minorities) and a managerial caste (made up for the most part of white majority males). In this acceptance of heteronomous work, women prostitute their own autonomy and men sacrifice their own wholeness and integrity. Women's work is divided from the power to shape and order that work; men's work is separated into a narrow, abstract sphere of "fiat" without feedback. She exalts her trivial state; he trivializes his humanity. Like many women who do not work, the career "servant girl" reduces her appreciation of and pleasure in her work to a single utilitarian motive—the job of being "needed."

If part of the attraction of the "Girl Friday" role is the vicarious participation in the life of the boss, the average secretary or clerical employee discovers that her usefulness is a brief and fragile commodity. "Planned obsolescence" applies to office workers as well as Chevrolets. One of the unwritten, often unspoken canons of the corporate world, "A girl who isn't likely to get married and leave wouldn't fit in around here," is a fact of life. Typing and steno pools, secretaries or dental assistants, the requirements are the same: mobile, sexy, efficient, friendly, and above all, not-likely-to-be-around-long-enough-to-be-concerned-about-vertical-mobility. It is precisely this quality of disposability and vulnerability that has led some corporations to exploit the feminist emphasis on work outside the home. Manpower executives make deliberate appeals to housewives to join the "temporary work force." As more than one observer has pointed out, not only are housewives useful to business as low-paid labor, but emergence from the household creates new consumer demands: "The system is adaptable enough to sell the working housewife a second car to get her to the office, expensive clothes, prepackaged foods to take the place of money-saving traditional cooking, household gadgets, children's summer camps . . . Also, a two-job family has more to spend."[22] The problem of women and work is not going to be solved by seducing bored housewives out of their suburban homes. It may even add to the pyramid of exploitable and alienated persons in our society:

> The new glorification of work and achievement that has replaced the old glorification of marriage and family in our women's

> magazines seems to me to contain the exact same seeds of unreality. So-called glamorous workers in so-called glamorous jobs will never account for more than a fraction of the work force in our most unglamorous job market. Only 15 per cent of women are classified as professionals, and most are teachers and nurses.[23]

If a woman can afford to reject the dubious allurements of the "pool" and the clerical maintenance caste, what can she do for meaningful work? Many women turn to volunteer work. Conduct manuals for "ladies" in the early industrial era commonly recommended philanthropy and volunteerism as a solution to female ennui, but often beneath the apparent concern for women's feelings of uselessness there were other societal motives. Moreover, time donated to charity was treated as an extension of the civilizing and nurturing function of women. While it was invested with the trappings of motherhood, it was, in reality, a form of social housekeeping. The human detritus and by-products of the male success machine had to be cared for by someone, and so it fell to woman's lot. A book on the *Duties of the Female Sex* from 1801, for example, stresses the obligation of wives of tradesmen and merchants to benefit in whatever way they could the families of the workmen employed by their husbands.

Thus, much female volunteer work (and women do most of it in our culture) is an act of complicity.

> If the Ladies can be counted on to help out, pitch in, clean up, and keep the lid on, there is no need for the Gentlemen in power to alter anything. Daughters of wealth, daughters of poverty; each do volunteer work as mothers and wives; and each volunteer to help the churches, schools, hospitals, medical researchers, politicians and museums raise money to maintain or expand their empires.
>
> Of course, the daughters of wealth can perform the volunteer labor of maintaining the status quo in more glamorous ways than the daughters of poverty can. But each woman is doing her share of maintaining things as they are. Each is compliant, in some way, in helping men insure the "triumph of conservatism": the enslavement, of class to class, race to race, and sex to sex.[24]

For most women it is easier to be concerned for a few significant "others" than it is to be concerned about themselves or about attempting to challenge power centers and structures that create the problems that volunteerism seeks to palliate. Once again, a woman's work motive is reduced to "being needed"—her moral power is diluted in activity that is cut off from transcendent action. She works because of a heteronomous imperative. Or she is immersed in purely narcissistic motives—she licks stamps for politicians for the privilege of sharing in the excitement of a campaign, or she answers telephone calls at the hunger center out of a sense of class guilt, or she types at the church center just to get out of the home for a while.

Volunteer work, thus, is often counterproductive in two ways. School systems, cultural institutions and community agencies that can depend on an undepleted reservoir of non-threatening volunteer help are likely to be sluggish about developing the priorities and structural changes that are necessary for real impact and extended community responsibility. On the individual level, volunteer work too often promotes a subjective, therapeutic motive for work among women, reducing public service to the same level as pursuits of diversion and self-expression like weaving and ballet classes, or gardening and handwriting analysis. Each of these activities can be pursued for its own sake, but many women pursue them for the wrong motive—they become a reflection of personal neuroses and insecurity rather than a product of true creative élan. Activities pursued for primarily therapeutic reasons are in the long run self-destructive for they are fundamentally private acts, onanistic and sterile, bringing little self-respect since they do not engage the larger human context beyond the self.

The therapeutic quality of much "volunteer service" is self-defeating. Its heteronomous quality is perhaps even more destructive. Particularly when it is rationalized with lofty religious motives, it is susceptible to translation into a kind of masochism: "There is nothing lower than being the servant of the servant of the sacred; in that world, every stirring of self-definition is guilt-ridden, shameful."[25] Volunteerism has been surrounded with an ideology that reinforces the myth of women's superior moral sensitivity, a quality that supposedly makes them uniquely suited to serve as "the unpaid conscience of the nation." To the extent that it absorbs jobs that would otherwise be part of the labor market, it not only exploits middle-class women's naïve altruism, but also lower-class working women who must work in order to survive.

The negative aspects are evident. But there is something potentially liberating in the concept of a group that is not "owned" by either government or business, that is not thrall to any political, religious or commercial interest. The non-paid volunteer is a potentially powerful catalyst, a free agent in the halls of Mammon. If women can find significant ways to enlarge their policy-making roles within the ambience of volunteer work, they may indeed do a great service to society. The platform of the National Organization of Women makes a pertinent distinction between volunteerism "for service" (activities that serve to maintain women's dependent and auxiliary status) and volunteerism "for change" (activities that lead to more active participation in decision-making processes in all private and public domains). Obviously, the latter represents an opportunity for women to engage in significant and meaningful work, work that can be an expression of personal autonomy as well as theonomous transcendence, an engagement with reality and time on a level that redeems both.

Alone, women will accomplish very little. Together, whether they are unpaid volunteers or underpaid office workers, they can begin the work of transforming the conditions of work in our society. Overcoming passivity, envy and envy avoidance, feelings of self-pity and inferiority, women are discovering the political effectiveness of bonding and banding together. The graffiti in women's lavatories have taken on a new assertiveness: "Raises, not roses!" "Make policy, not coffee!" "Don't agonize, organize!" Coal miners today, but secretaries and clerks tomorrow. Cinderella is rising up out of the ashes!

> Truthfully I can say this is one of the happiest times of my life and one of the fullest times of my life. I always say, "Death, *man,* you can come anytime because I feel that I'm really whole. I feel like I can fit into anything, that I can *do* anything, that I can go *anywhere* and *be* anything." And therefore there's nothing I have to prove. I've already done it. And I feel so good about it, because I *chose* what I wanted to be. I chose it. And I *got* it! And *that's* what makes me feel so good!
>
> —Sophenia Maxwell, Electrical Mechanic, quoted in *Conversations: Working Women Talk About Doing a Man's Job*

Much has been said and written about women and "the fear of success." In anatomizing this phenomenon it is important to recognize that the fear of success is rooted in the fear of failure as well as in envy avoidance. Women are accustomed and conditioned to being judged on their personal characteristics—on the basis of what they are, how they behave—rather than on the basis of what they can do, what they are capable of accomplishing. Erica Jong, a contemporary poet and novelist puts the "success" problem in concrete terms:

> Just about the most common complaint of talented women . . . is that they can't finish things. Partly because finishing things implies being judged—but also because finishing things means being grown up. More important, it means possibly succeeding at something. And success, for women, is always partly failure.[26]

Fear of being judged, fear of autonomy—fear of having to assume responsibility for what one does—is the root of the success problem. Because of their "other-centered" conditioning, it is difficult for many women to focus on a goal other than pleasing someone's (everyone's) expectations. It is easier to conform to an "image" than to initiate and accomplish a task. Even women who have attained success continue to have problems with "drift" and often lack long-range career strategy. The drive, the persistence, the goal-centeredness is lacking. Women typically do not internalize the identity of a doer, a worker, to the extent that men do, and thus may lack momentum in a lifework.

The experience of black women presents a significant contrast to this picture. Research generally indicates that black women professionals exhibit more "survival" capability than their counterparts in the white middle class. Assertiveness qualities are higher, initiative and momentum over the long haul are more consistent, dependency on mentors and husbands is lower, and in general self-sufficiency traits are much more developed. Studies indicate that women from white immigrant families are more likely to share these traits. Competence is not necessarily the crucial factor. According to one study:

> The thread that connected them was the fact that they had to work. That is, the economic rationale—the most legitimate in American Society—gave them the answer to the question that all women face: "Why aren't you at home, and aren't you denying your family something by not being there?"[27]

Black women, and many first-generation American women, have an inherited or conditioned sense of themselves as workers. In the case of the black woman, her role as a stabilizing force and provider in the black community for several generations has given her a strength and resourcefulness—a confidence and a sticking power, a success capability—that many middle-class white women lack.

Women's tendency to fuse the need to achieve with the need to affiliate will sometimes place them in situations in which they are likely to be exempted from the normal disciplines and performance hurdles that apply to men. Their success, therefore, can often be ambiguous when they are rewarded for the wrong reasons: "Women are often seduced into a type of high commitment by rewards directed at their sex status . . . rather than their occupational status."[28] Likewise, a woman's fear of competition, like her fear of being judged, may exclude her from the normal *rites de passage* that lead to success. A woman's inability to express annoyance and criticism, her timidity in expressing praise or enjoyment, her inability to say "No," to take risks and initiate action will limit her in the give and take of competitive situations. As we have noted before, insecure, egobound, envious people cannot rise above petty suspicions and hurts, they ignore rather than confront others, or find ways of manipulating them to achieve their ends. These are among the greatest obstacles that face women who have embarked on a "success" trajectory. Many women deprived of the tools and temperament necessary for competitive interchange, retreat to a protected status. In effect, they "castle" themselves under the aegis of a male mentor or within a protected enclave of peers; some may set themselves apart by adopting adjunct or marginal status. They never really play in the game, hence they are never really taken seriously.

One of the most important tools women require for acceptance in work roles is mastery of the language of power. Robin Lakoff has described "women's language," with its characteristic vocabulary, tendency to vacuous adjectives, intensifiers, question intonations, subjunctives and qualifying adverbs, as a "language of deference." The effect of deferential language is to establish the speaker as one not responsible for being truthful and being right. Syntactically, lexically and phonologically, women's language allows them to abdicate from judgment, decision, choice. It presupposes a certain "powerlessness" in the one who asserts, a distancing from responsibility.[29] Happily, this genteel survival of the Victorian era is declining, particularly among the young. But the residue is still an inhibiting factor for many women who want to embark on a serious career effort. The change is evident in some of our contemporary women writers and politicians who have mastered the male style of bombast and sexual hyperbole. Women who exploit the male idiom, however, run the risk of perpetuating the very "macho," patriarchal structures of interrelationship which an androcentric language supports. Perhaps, as with sex roles, there is a happy medium—an androgynous language—appropriate for all seasons, all sexes, that avoids extreme deference as much as exploitation and relies on the candor of "Yes for yes, and no for no."

A variety of other behaviors in women reflect a fear of power. Body language is as crucial as speech. Clothing that reassures male colleagues that one is not a threat, avoidance of eye contact and touching, contraction rather than extension of the body, smiling. The ubiquitous feminine smile, for example, has been compared to "the Uncle Tom shuffle"—a gesture of submission and accommodation, of desire for approval.

Women speak about money and power as they speak about sex: in modest, cautionary tones. Women seek money and power as they seek sex: generally in moderation, somewhat apologetically, without ecstatic abandon. They have learned the lessons at their mother's knee all too well: "no excess" and "no excelling." Above all, they have learned that power or money sought for its own sake, like work loved for its own sake, is somehow tainted, a betrayal of one's nature.

> Women are supposed to feel the same way about sex as they do about money. Traditionally, women are not supposed to say they want to *make* money or *make* sex. It is something that women are not supposed to do, or are not supposed to say they do. Sex or money is something that is supposed to "happen" to women . . .
>
> Female inherited *wealth* is somehow "invisible" and, as such, is not threatening. Women *working* for cash, or having to, is as vulgar and embarrassing to our traditional minds as is the sight of a woman exposing a bank roll at a dinner table.[30]

Making money is a supreme act of personal power in our society. To reject the opportunity to make money out of fear, inertia or guilt is to sacrifice an important source of autonomy and commitment. To reject the opportunity to make money for other transcendent motives may also be a supreme act of autonomy. Of this we will say more later.

Women have begun to disbelieve the old myths about their power as women. They know now where real power lies, and they are consciously, calculatingly seeking it. They know, too, that the first obstacles to be overcome are those within themselves. The authors of *The Managerial Woman* list the most prominent psychological barriers:

> 1. Women describe themselves as waiting to be chosen—discovered, invited, persuaded, asked to accept a promotion.
> 2. Women describe themselves as hesitant, as waiting to be told what to do.
> 3. Women describe themselves as often feeling conflicted and confused about their own goals.
> 4. Women say that they become extremely anxious when they have to deal with unknowns.
> 5. Women say that they find criticism difficult to deal with.
> 6. Women describe themselves as reluctant to take risks.
> 7. Women often say that the only way they can deal with their feelings of guilt over having a career is to try to be a perfect woman/wife/mother simultaneously.[31]

Once these hang-ups are overcome, reconciled, there are other traps to be avoided: professional elitism, the "superwoman" role, the "queen bee" scenario (making others play Cinderella among the ashes). Worst of all, perhaps, is the obvious possibility that women who have achieved power will be co-opted by the system and use it in the same ways men always have. Will there be a female Watergate somewhere down the road? And no doubt some women, in the euphoria of their newly acquired opportunities, will fall victim to the "Peter Principle" and flaunt their incompetence in high places. "Readiness is all," and women should discern their moment wisely.

Is Cinderella ready to wear the fragile and transparent slipper of power? She should not go naïvely into her new kingdom. Her very appearance is a catalyst for change; women in the halls of power are harbingers of conflict. Every woman on the rise will be a sign of contradiction. The new feminist myths that describe the placid vistas of unlimited opportunity now open to women are Pollyannic dreams. If a woman would prepare herself for achievement, for success, she must prepare herself for conflict. Her socialization and pacifist temperament will resist this. She may even try to ignore the hostility that her most innocent gestures and decisions may provoke. Misogyny is deeply rooted in our culture and will surface most brutishly in the face of emerging female power and autonomy. It is found not only in men, but in women.

More importantly, the task of "social housekeeping," in which women were relied upon to comfort the cries of the disadvantaged, will be abandoned for the more crucial tasks of policy making and reshaping the very structures of society. The conflicts that were covert will be exposed.

> As women seek self-definition and self-determination, they will, perforce illuminate, on a broad new scale, the existence of conflict as a basic process of existence. As long as women were used in a massive attempt to suppress certain fundamental human conflicts, the basic process of conflict itself remained obscure . . . women are not creating conflict; they are exposing the fact that conflict exists.
>
> . . . when women feel in conflict, there is a good reason to believe they should be in conflict. This, at least, can help at the start. Women's energies and hopes will not be drained before they even begin to accumulate. In the past, women lived under a framework of conceptions and prescriptions that was destructive of them. They were attempting to fit themselves into a model of behavior that did not fit anyone; then they blamed themselves if they could not squeeze into it, or if they felt conflicted in the process.[32]

The contemporary woman will have to learn how to manage conflict in a productive way: conflict with husbands and children, with bosses and subordinates, with vested interests. Above all, she will have to contend with a new self-image and the indestructible residue of the old feminine mystique. She will accept the challenge of a life lived in a creative tension, rather than the "sell-out" proposed by *The Total Woman*—the heroism of the damned. She will discover that conflict is not so much the ultimate test of love as a supreme expression of it, of a profound sense of caring about everything and everyone—including herself.

> I am a wife, a mother, a businesswoman. My husband sums up my situation in a little story he tells. He says, "How in the world can you watch the metal market fluctuate up and down, make or lose thousands of dollars in a day's time without batting an eyelash? But you break down and cry a heap of tears because it's the night of a P.T.A. meeting and you have a runner in your nylon hose!" That is my life in a nutshell.
>
> —Grace Smith Whately, Chairperson of the Board of Universal Investments, Inc. and several other firms, quoted in *Conversations: Working Women Talk About Doing a Man's Job*

In the conclusion of the fairy tale, Cinderella goes off to the palace with her Prince, presumably to live the life of the Leisured Lady, happily ever after. There was a time when any woman would aspire to such a life, but no more. The insistent chimes of "Midnight" still announce the double desire of every woman's heart; the necessity of meaningful work, and the need for meaningful relationships. How long must the day be divided ruthlessly into two halves—half for work, half for relationships? How long must women lead a double life, work a double shift? Can Life and Work converge?

Some women have found a magic amalgam, usually through a service or creative profession that permits greater control over one's time, more contact hours at home where personal life and occupational tasks can be carried out simultaneously. Rosemary Ruether describes her typical day:

> Herc, my husband, goes to American University (Methodist), and I go east to Howard University. At noon most of us come home again for lunch. Then everybody leaves again but myself and Mimi. Mimi colors and plays and I read. Sometimes I read in warm baths. I also think and write. Thinking and writing takes place in various postures. I do a lot of cleaning while I am thinking. Think, think (scrub, scrub), type, type, type . . .
>
> It is difficult for me to find that part of my daily activities which can be called "my work," because there is really no such special activity which can be disentangled from the pattern of our lives in general. When I am teaching a class, it is not a special ac-

> tivity which I do as "work," but is simply one extension of what I am. Other extensions of what I am include children, houses, reading, writing, running a catechetical program for an Episcopal church, making banners to carry on peace marches and illegal liturgical processions . . .
>
> I have never felt so rushed that I couldn't spend an evening lying on the floor with Becky, David and Mimi watching "Pollyanna."[33]

Elsewhere Ruether has commented on the destructive effects that capitalism and socialism (Marxist) have had on the household. If capitalism has isolated the home and the woman at its center, socialism has co-opted woman into a male concept of alienated work, "leaving the home little more than a bedroom and a nucleus of fleeting personal relations. As one function after another is collectivised outside the family, the family progressively loses its self-determination and becomes totally determined by social forces over which it has no power." Socialists as well as feminists must rethink and resocialize the home "by bringing access to work and political decision making back into a more integral relationship to it."[34]

We would all like to be able to say, "My life and my work are one." At the moment, this happy convergence of home and work is for the most part a luxury of a certain class of professionals. They can accomplish the "merger" without changing structures. Most women will not be so lucky.

The dilemma of "Midnight" is not unlike the dilemma of androgyny. How does one salvage the best of both roles—masculine and feminine—the best of both worlds—home and work—in a meaningful paradigm, a personal blueprint? It is obvious that if women and their families are to survive, the structures of labor in our society will have to be adjusted, adapted, changed (working hours, child-care facilities, parental leaves, etc.). It is also obvious that significant changes will have to be made in the traditional structure of roles in the family. Husbands and wives may have to accept a modified living standard and qualify their ambitions if both partners are to enjoy total participation in the project of existence.

Women, in resolving to work, should perhaps also resolve:

1. Not to work anywhere without trying to reshape the conditions of that work in some way, and
2. Not to leave home without enlisting others—spouse, chil-

dren, friends—in the care-giving, hearth-making functions that are the common task of humanity.

The primitive bifurcations of the "Midnight" syndrome must be overcome. Denise Levertov's "Prayer for Revolutionary Love" is not a fairy tale, it is a real-life scenario:

> That a woman not ask a man to leave meaningful work to follow her.
>
> That a man not ask a woman to leave meaningful work to follow him.
>
> That no one try to put Eros in bondage.
> But that no one put a cudgel in the hands of Eros.
>
> That our loyalty to one another and our loyalty to our work not be set in false conflict.
>
> That our love for each other give us love for each other's work.
> That our love for each other's work give us love for one another.
>
> That our love for each other's work give us love for one another.
> That our love for each other give us love for each other's work.
>
> That our love for each other, if need be,
> give way to absence. And the unknown.
>
> That we endure absence, if need be,
> without losing our love for each other,
> Without closing our doors to the unknown.[35]

the legend

For Goldilocks there is no happy ending—from failure to find what is fitting for her, she awakes as if from a bad dream, and runs away.

Goldilocks' story illustrates the meaning of the difficult choice the child must master: is he to be like father, like mother, or like child? To decide who he wants to be in respect to these basic human positions is indeed a tremendous psychological battle, an ordeal every human being has to undergo. But while the child is not yet ready to be in Father's or Mother's place, just accepting that of the child is no solution—this is why the three tests are not sufficient. For growth, realization that one is still a child must be coupled with another recognition: that one has to become oneself, something different from either parent, or from being merely their child.

—Bruno Bettelheim, *The Uses of Enchantment*[1]

Being single is not really anything I think about except that it's obviously a part of my state of being, and when I think of myself, it's one characteristic that defines me. But I feel single and tribal. That is, since I've grown up I'm always looking for family—kinfolk and family are not necessarily the same thing.

—Elizabeth Ashley, in *Three Women Alone*[2]

The moral of the story is that people are not animals, that Culture is not Nature. But the honey is the same as Goldilocks; she enters the story when the bears leave to seek her, and she leaves the story in her human form when the bears bring her back in her natural one. Thus Goldilocks and Honey are . . . homologous in their color and sweetness in their structural position as singletons, and in their functional roles as mediators between the cultural and the natural.

—Eugene Hammel, "Levi-Strauss and the Three Bears"[3]

Goldilocks is an impostor. For several generations this bedtime favorite has masqueraded as a fairy tale, when in reality it is a moral fable. The story lacks certain characteristic features of a fairy tale, most notably the expected happy ending. In this tale the heroine ends as she began: There is neither recovery nor consolation; there is no resolution of conflict.

The cautionary significance of the tale is especially evident in its earliest version—believed to be an ancient Scottish tale of three bears that are intruded upon by a she-fox. The original version, *Scrapefoot,* is probably a survival of an old beast epic or the "Reynard the Fox" cycle. Another early version substitutes a shrewish old woman for the fox. The emphasis in both these tales is on the vindictive response of the bears to the intrusion: the fox is thrown out the window (after being threatened with hanging and drowning), and the old woman is thrown onto the church steeple (after being threatened with burning and drowning). The moral is clear: don't invade others' privacy and keep hands off private property.

This proprietary theme gives the tale a quality of modernity, and in fact, it is a comparatively recent arrival in narrative literature. Southey's *Three Bears* of 1836 (with the old woman as intruder) is the earliest printed version. A critical point in its evolution occurs in 1872 with the publication of the first version in which the intruder is a girl named "Silverhair" (later "Goldenhair" then "Goldenlocks"), and the bears are fully and explicitly a family.

The significance of these two narrative elements is crucial to the meaning of the fable. The appearance of "golden hair" in a folk or fairy tale always signifies a capacity for spiritualization. Material gold (in the form of apples, feathers, furs, straw) is often contrasted sharply with this finer ore of the spirit, always associated with a hero or heroine. The golden hair symbolizes the inner world of human talents and values and its capacity to transform brute nature into "soul." In the earliest tales the bears had been undifferentiated as to sex and relationship, although it is often implied that they are all male. Significantly, the family constellation and the appearance of the golden-haired girl-heroine are linked chronologically with the apotheosis of the Victorian cult of domesticity. The child-woman is a kind of spiritual emblem of the period, and the family is often portrayed as a highly structured moral sanctuary. Thus, Papa, Mama and Baby Bear appear in folk literature, significantly, at a time when the nuclear family is in the ascendancy as a hallowed haven.

Historically, as the story is replicated at the turn of the century, the thematic emphasis shifts from the bears to Goldilocks. Instead of a tale focused on a familial-tribal response to intrusion, it becomes more and more the story of a highly individuated intruder. As a "singleton," Goldilocks is an archetypal symbol of the twentieth-century personality: a transient, highly mobile, self-actualized consumer. She comes from nowhere, she has no story to tell. (In contrast to the dwarfs in *Snow White,* the bears are not overwhelmed by her beauty or moved by her tale of woe.)

Her elaboration in the story parallels a developing theme of "sweetness." Honey is first mentioned in an 1889 version; the mixing of a sweetener in the porridge as a deliberate act occurs first in 1947. By the early 1960s most versions of the tale present a highly elaborated structural role for honey. Goldilocks' behavior changes analogously. In the early versions, her uninvited intrusion is regarded as a hostile act (although her entrance seems less malicious in intent than that of her predecessors, the fox and the old woman). As time goes on, she becomes "sweeter" and "sweeter"—at first just lost and confused, then indifferent, finally ingenuous. At the same time, the bears gradually take on a Walt Disney aspect. By 1924 there are expressions of desire for further contact between the bears and the intruder; by 1928 Goldilocks invites the bears to tea, and in 1955 Goldilocks and her mother have the bears over for breakfast. Hammel sums up the historical symbolism of the tale:

> A good deal of the change in style and focus seems to parallel developments in the society to which Goldilocks belongs. Where the

> older versions conjure up visions of a strict, proper, and somewhat stuffy world, like that of Mary Poppins, the later ones are set squarely in an American suburb. If this kind of stylistic change continues, we may expect to see versions with Goldilocks and Baby Bear trotting off to school together, and Papa Bear going bowling with a newly invented Mr. Goldilocks. Some socially conscious author will, no doubt, turn the story of the evil intruder and her noble animal hosts into a parable of race relations, and we may even see Goldilocks and Baby Bear being bused to school. Myth, as Lowie observed, is more the story of its authors than of its subject.[4]

This amelioration in the role of Goldilocks and her graduate rapprochement with the bears seems to highlight an underlying social imperative: the necessity of confrontation with the radical "other," and the subsequent process of integrating the "other" into one's own existence and being. Thus, on one level, the historical evolution of the tale reflects the contemporary trend away from nucleated sameness, inwardness and exclusivity in the structure of relationships and toward modes of affiliation that reflect openness, availability and variety.

On a more personal and psychological level, Goldilocks is a parable of role experimentation and the search for identity. The constellation of the bears has an uncanny similarity to the structure of ego states in the theory of transactional analysis: the Parent selves, judgmental, critical, demanding or nurturing; the Child self, self-indulgent and irresponsible compliant and passive, or manipulative and instinctive. (Significantly, the appearance of Papa Bear, Mama Bear and Baby Bear came just a few years prior to Freud's elaboration of his theory of the triadic structure of the personality into superego, ego and id.)

The developing personality must experiment with many roles, with various modes of relating to others, then discard the ill-fitting masks and scenarios in order to create an original self. Goldilocks is initially "lost in the forest," an archetypal symbol expressing the "need to find oneself." She tries on all of the bear-personas for size. Her experience is analogous to that of her fictional cousin, *Alice in Wonderland*. Alice alternately takes potions to shrink herself, then enlarge herself—struggling to find just the right size for her circumstances, just the right role to mediate her encounters.

Finally, Goldilocks consumes Baby Bear's porridge (which suits her taste), she sits in his chair (which breaks under her weight) and she falls asleep in his bed (which she finds more comfortable than the others). Only the child's role fits. Ultimately she is discovered. Like many of her real-life sisters, Goldilocks stands accused of an act of regression, of abdication from autonomy, of sin—"a refusal to become conscious," to take responsibility for her own life.

> Goldilocks' experience in the bears' house at least teaches her that regression to infantilism offers no escape from the difficulties of growing up. Becoming oneself, the story suggests, is a process begun by sorting out what is involved in one's relations to one's parents.[5]

Appropriately, in the end, she must return to the forest, to a condition of essential solitude, shorn of her addictions and dependencies, responsible for her self. Aloneless is her destiny. Intimacy must always be transcended; it is necessary to begin again, and again, and again.

The story of Goldilocks also juxtaposes the values of nature and culture. Or, put another way, the tale contrasts that which is determined for us with that which we must determine for ourselves. We, like Goldilocks, draw energy and sustenance from our insertion into a "natural" role—but in the end we, too, realize we don't belong there. Biology and the blind rule of custom are not our destiny:

> It is senseless . . . to describe our prevailing male-female arrangements as "natural." They are of course a part of nature, but if they should contribute to the extinction of our species, that fact would be part of nature, too. Our impulse to change these arrangements is as natural as they are, and more compatible with our survival on earth . . .
>
> The quintessential feature of human life, along with its pervasive inner instability and stress, is its self-creating nature: its control—for better or for worse—over the direction in which it develops . . .
>
> We are what we have made ourselves, and we must continue to make ourselves as long as we exist at all.[6]

If we assume that Goldilocks simply barged into the wrong house, and that some day she will find one where she fits—then she remains an unfinished person, one who never learns, one who must constantly undergo the same initiation, affiliation, transference, always on the verge of wholeness and happiness. But if we prefer to read the story in a more dynamic sense, Goldilocks emerges as a unique symbol of transcendence among fairy-tale heroines. Her return to the forest is the source of her strength. No single relationship is sufficient in itself to complete her life. She returns to the essential solitude that is the basis of autonomous relationship, the solitude that is a principle of mediation between intimacy and privacy, role and identity, affiliation and self-actualization, nature and culture.

Goldilocks is at home in the forest.

FOUR

Goldilocks and the Search for the Perfect Family

MOST people are convinced of the truth of Martin Buber's maxim, "All real living is *meeting*." And yet, increasingly in the contemporary era, these relationships, these affiliations which seem so necessary, become the chief obstacles to full human development. Some go so far as to say that the primary affiliation, the family, "has become, in this century, the ultimately perfected form of *non-meeting*."

One thing is certain, that for everyone—men as well as women—personal development and psychological growth progress only by means of affiliation. Autonomy requires relationship and at the same time makes it posible to transcend its limitations. Relationship makes it possible to believe in others in a way that confirms one's faith in oneself. Human communion is, thus, the basis of authentic theonomy: a condition of existence in which self-sufficiency and self-righteousness compromise with self-transcendence and contingency, in which the individual achieves a relation of equilibrium with all that is, and with the ground of Being itself. The project of existence is the creation of this eco-self.

For women, the task is complicated by a characteristic ambiguity. Women are typically more socialized to the necessity for affiliation, more prepared in terms of conviction as well as interpersonal skills to find fulfillment in relationships. Men, from their earliest years, are weaned away from dependence on attachments and learn to find their fulfillment in enterprise, achievement, adulation. The kind of relationship they require is, so often, not one of mutuality but a one-sided, disproportionate need for ego reinforcement.

The value that women place on interpersonal relationships and their exceptional capacity for achieving affiliation places them in a double bind. If, like many men, they choose not to build their lives around one meaningful relationship, they are considered abnormal. If they should choose to do so, they often overrelate and transform their male partner—or in the absence of marriage, a loved one—into a larger-than-life image of the ultimate One who can meet all of their needs, and whose needs they presume to be totally adequate to supply. So often the woman who loves abdicates from responsibility for her own confirmation by expecting and demanding that affirmation from the significant other person in her life. The other-centered, approval-seeking reflexes of feminine socialization condition a woman to "feel right" only when whatever she does is done for that significant Other. We have noted before the inordinate demands that this often places on the woman's partner or children and the absolute, exclusive bond, the continuous reassurance that it extracts. In a sense, it inverts the normal pattern of satisfaction in the human personality.

Prince Charming, The Expected One, exists only as a correlative projection of Sleeping Beauty, Snow White and Cinderella. As woman emerges from her existential sleep and subservience, the significant Other is refracted into a spectrum of lovers, friends, husbands. The loved one is essentially multiple, a network of meaningful relationships and/or a lover who is protean enough to play the multiple roles that a dynamic relationship requires. There is no "total woman" because there is no "total man."

Women's expectations in regard to conjugal partners have been radically altered by the change in their own status. No more than 16 per cent of American families currently conform to the typical stereotype with a father supporting a non-working mother and their children. Fifty per cent of all American women are now in the labor force and almost half of those are "women alone": widowed, divorced or separated from their husbands, or single women who have never been married. A woman's identity is no longer circumscribed by motherhood, child rearing, and wifely duties. She has, in fact, been emancipated from the narrow and constricting social imperative that limited her to "woman's sphere."

This loss of a clearly defined social role has given many women a new sense of identity and existential space. For some women, however, it has been a cause of confusion and anomie, of paralysis in the face of unanticipated options. In either case, it has made the choice of a life companion even more crucial. Where will the "new woman" find a "new man" who is equal to the shifting roles that personal autonomy may require? Expectations are necessarily higher; the demands on a mate intensified. The discovery and exploration of alternative selves, a necessary component of autonomy, may leave one's partner confused and frustrated. Can the institution of marriage and family—as we have known it—sustain what some sociologists are now calling a "quantum leap" in the evolution of its structure?

Women are caught in a time lapse between the old and the new. Their changing self-image and emerging autonomy have been the catalyst for a universal crisis in social structures:

> The age in which we live is shivering amidst the tremors of ontological breakdown . . . The moral mandates, the structural givens, the standard brand governments, religions, economics, the very consensual reality is breaking down, the underlying fabric of life and process by which we organized our reality and thought we knew who and why and where we are. The world by which we understood ourselves, a world which began in its essential mandates two thousand years ago with certain premises about man, God, reality, and the moral and metaphysical order, and which in terms of our existential lives began about 300 years ago with the scientific revolution; is a world that no longer works, whose lease has run out, whose paradigms are eroding, and that no longer provides us with the means and reference points by which we understand ourselves. We are not unlike the cartoon cat who runs off the cliff and keeps on running, treading air over the abyss before he discovers his predicament and says, "Oops!"
>
> . . . There is a lag between the end of an age and the discovery of that end. We are the children of the lag . . .[7]

There are no scripts and no models for the new age. Marriage and the family will, no doubt, remain the primary locus of relationships—but the exclusivity, division of roles, and permanence of these relationships will be qualified and, in some cases, radically altered. Many more, perhaps, will seek a more explicit expression of personal autonomy in the single life.

Like the mythic figure of Eurydice, we will be tempted by nostalgic and pleading voices to turn back to the security of the old roles, but to succumb is to immobilize not only one's own soul, but society itself.

> We have ritualized security. Our mistake was that we didn't break away from the beginning and create something in our own terms.
>
> —Marianne, in Ingmar Bergman's *Scenes from a Marriage*

"All happy families resemble one another, but each unhappy family is unhappy in its own way." The opening sentence from Tolstoy's *Anna Karenina* underscored the novel's theme: deviance from the accepted norm in social relationships will bring unhappiness. It was a theme appropriate to an era and a social class characterized by a rigid conception of domestic hierarchies and protocols.

Today, an inversion of Tolstoy's maxim might be a more accurate reflection of the contemporary scene. It is, in fact, in the "typical" families, the ones most closely modeled on the "norm," where unhappiness is rampant. This suggests that the problems allied to marriage and family in this era are not problems of deviance from the norm, but of adherence to it. The stresses, the breakdowns, have a structural rather than personal origin.

But we resist admitting that there may be something wrong with the fundamental structures of marriage and family. We prefer to view these problems as personal and idiosyncratic, and therefore responsive to therapeutic solutions. Women, especially, have been vulnerable to the guilt that is projected when social dislocations occur, as when working mothers are blamed for family disintegration or frigid wives for marital infidelity. We prefer to find a scapegoat, to identify some expression of individual deviance rather than recognize an inherent flaw in the structure of the marriage-bond or the family itself. "Band-Aids" rather than major surgery are recommended. We seek therapy: marital counseling, psychic self-help programs, conflict management, sibling dynamics, assertiveness training, parenting classes.

Indeed, if we were to admit that there is something inherently disjointed, fundamentally wrong, with the family, we threaten the entire fabric of social intercourse and the political order itself. The scenarios and scripts that prevail in the larger arenas of civilization are learned in its cradle—the family. As the primordial paradigm of all institutional systems, the family is the key to change, whether it be by revolution or evolution.

Sociologists have noted the steady drift of familial structure toward the "symmetrical family," a primary unit in which division of roles along sexual lines is at a minimum. In our own era working wives commonly share the provider role with husbands, but inevitably work a "double shift" because husbands are not sharing the home and child-care duties. But most sociologists expect the trend to continue. The force of feminism as well as inflation is likely to accelerate this gradual convergence of man's and woman's worlds.

> In this century wives have been doing a job outside the home that they did not greatly care for and the husbands a minor job inside the home that they did not greatly care for either . . . By the next century—with the pioneers of 1970 already at the front of the column—society will have moved from a) one demanding job for the wife and one for the husband, through b) two demanding jobs for the wife and one for the husband, to c) two demanding jobs for the wife and two for the husband. The symmetry will be complete. Instead of two jobs there will be four.
>
> Such a new relationship to the world outside the home will affect all that goes on in it, and vice versa. "If we have children," more wives will say, "will you look after them as much as I?" And, "If my career requires a move of house, will that count as much as yours?"
>
> . . . Strains will be inescapable. There will inevitably be more divorces because people will be seeking a more multi-faceted adjustment to each other, with the two outside jobs clicking with the two inside ones; and because the task will be harder, there will be more failures.[8]

The advantages of this symmetrical arrangement for promoting female autonomy are evident. The sociological impetus is soundly based and has a momentum of its own. But many will ask, is the change ultimately in the best interests of men, women and children; of society as a whole?

A recent and provocative answer to this question has been proposed by Dorothy Dinnerstein, a psychologist. In her book *The Mermaid and the Minotaur,* Dinnerstein proposes that a primary cause of the personal, social and political neuroses that characterize contemporary life is the female monopoly of early child care. Of course, it is nothing new to blame our social ills on "momism." What is unique about Dinnerstein's thesis is that she locates the problem in the *structure* of child-care arrangements, not necessarily in the quality of the care.

The fact that human infants receive more or less exclusive and unconditional care from a female seduces them into fantasies and expectations that are inevitably shattered, crushed—"fantasies of a world that automatically obeys, even anticipates their wishes." With the expectations generated by intense mothering (or, in the absence of it, belief that one has been cheated out of it) we manage to console ourselves for this trauma indirectly, through mastery, competence and enterprise. Successful activity provides some compensation for the lost joy of passive, effortless wish fulfillment. The fact that our earliest experience of power is that of an absolute female will is the basis of an inevitable reflex, an acceptance of paternal authority as a sanctuary from maternal tyranny: "as we leave infancy . . . the possibility of transferring dependent, submissive feeling to the second parent—whose different gender carries the promise of a new deal, a clean sweep—entices us into the trap of male domination."[9]

Moreover, the female monopoly of child care carries with it a whole universe of symbiotic and neurotic relations between mother-raised men and mother-raised women. The asymmetries of the personal experience are translated into the disjunctions of the public experience. The mother-raised society reveals a variety of disparate ills whose interrelationship Dinnerstein illuminates: Distortions appear not only in the exercise of power and submission to it, but in the compulsive drive for success and in the work syndrome, in attitudes toward death and toward the female body, in erotic relationships and in religious experience. Paradoxically, "the primitive cornerstone of human solidarity" is at the same time "the primitive cornerstone of human pathology." The long-range implications of Dinnerstein's analysis suggest that no fundamental change either in the relationship of men and women or in social structures can be achieved "without full male participation in early child care."[10]

The distortions that appear in erotic relationships are especially crucial and critical to any consideration of women's capacity for fulfillment with a life companion. Mother-raised men are likely to demand the same kind of ego-feeding care from their marriage partners that they received from their mothers. Since he is "apt to be the one who can more literally relive the infant experience of fulfilling primitive wishes through unqualified access to another body," he is likely to be more possessive. In mother-raised women, the capacity for vicarious experience is more dominant. Sexual spontaneity and aggressiveness in the female can too easily recall the absolute power of the mother in a male partner, therefore socialization tends to mute this capacity. She is apt to be engrossed more in being a source of pleasure rather than in giving herself over to pleasure. At the same time, she is less afraid of the dependency that physical and emotional intimacy implies, and of the access to the inner self that it provides:

> She can more readily re-evoke in him the unqualified, boundless, helpless passion of infancy. If he lets her, she can shatter his adult sense of power and control; she can bring out the soft, wild, naked baby in him.
>
> Men try to handle this danger with many kinds of sex-segregating institutions that they seem always and everywhere driven to create. Secret societies, hunting trips, pool parlors, wars —all of these provide men with sanctuary from the impact of women, with refuges in which they can recuperate from the temptation to give way to ferocious, voracious dependence, and recover their feelings of competence, autonomy, dignity.[11]

Thus, in the erotic relationship men and women repeat and relive, in interaction with the opposite sex, fundamental feelings that first take shape in the original infant-parent relation. No doubt these are not the only feelings that are relived, reinvented—but they do seem to be the most crucial. Time is running out on the argument that these distortions provide a "complementarity," a "*vive la difference*" which enhances love between men and women. In reality, the complementarity is a disguised neurotic symbiosis that perpetuates immaturity. It is a fragile relation, one that is hardly adequate to the growing demands of a symmetrical social order.

There is evidence, too, that the most destructive element in single-sex monopoly of child care is the degree of role specialization. Philip Slater has observed that boys identify most strongly with whichever parent is least extreme in the performance of his or her sex role. Other studies indicate that there is a strong negative correlation between sharp parental role specialization and the emotional health of children.[12] (These generalizations, of course, are mitigated by the example of families that are atypical in structure. In extended families, the effects of sharp specialization between the parents is diluted by the presence of parental substitutes. Perhaps also in single-parent families where one adult fulfills multiple roles, although this is a far more complex situation.)

For a woman the first step toward full personhood for herself, as well as for her children, is relinquishment of the one role that all others have often been sacrificed to: imperial motherhood. Dinnerstein puts it bluntly: "Mothering must become obsolete." "Parenting" must take its place. Some would argue that this flies in the face of biologically rooted differences between men and women, in terms of nurturing instincts. Dinnerstein and others would suggest that we have perhaps given disproportionate psychic weight to post-partum mammalian reflexes, and as a result have aggrandized a "myth of motherhood." At the same time we have minimized the distinctly human capacities that true parenting requires and the role of intentionality. Paradoxically, it is men who perhaps can best appreciate this dimension of parenthood. Precisely because he cannot carry the baby in his belly or suckle it at his breast, a father is more likely to be conscious of the intentional, voluntary aspect of parenthood. He assumes his role under less emotional and biological duress than a mother does.

As the father's contact with children increases, the more instinctive his attachment to them becomes. He can participate more in the involuntary aspect of parenting. Conversely, women who share parenting gain more opportunity to develop the voluntary, conscious aspect of human generation. Shared child-care arrangements permit mothers to experience the time they spend with children as a deliberate and voluntary option.

The present disenchantment with motherhood among American women should not be interpreted as evidence of "unnatural" feelings toward children. Rather, it is an indication that child care, not childbearing, is problematic. Women have begun to resent the burden of their exclusive role and have also begun to question (sometimes intuitively and unconsciously) the compulsive relations induced by the mother's role in our society. Men have begun to question their own exclusion and abdication from a primary role in early child care and the effect this has had on the male psyche. Most men, however, "are too enmeshed in the system to understand how it works and too

other major revolution in the meaning of human relationships within the social structure.

What we have previously described as the triptychal development of the spiritual personality from heteronomy through autonomy to theonomy has analogous patterns in the psycho-history of social structures. The heteronomic quality of the Old Testament as well as the feudal order is obvious. The individual exists only insofar as he/she is a component of a larger entity, a kinship structure, a "people," a nation. The archetypal spiritual personalities are those who solidify and personify these structures: Moses, Abraham, Jacob, David. In the second genesis after the flood, it is Noah and his sons who emerge as the archetypal progenitors, not Noah and his wife. Many of the narratives of the Old Testament are framed by familiar epithets placing a patriarchal figure in the context of a people, a role that gives him an identity larger than himself and a mission that comes from beyond himself: ". . . he was great among the Jews and popular with the multitude of his brethren, for he sought the welfare of his people and spoke peace to all his people" (Esther 10:3). Even the women, when they emerge from the shadow of the patriarchs, identify themselves with the fate and destiny of a tribe or nation: ". . . Your people shall be my people and your God my God" (Ruth 1:16). In the heteronomic era personality is not individuated in a conceptual way. There is a prevailing sense of being "incomplete" as an individual, of the necessity of identification with the center of power in the community.

This *dynastic* sense of polity (which perhaps survives in groups like the Mafia today) contrasts sharply with the *dyadic* sense which prevailed in the post-Renaissance and Reformation eras. The dyadic ethos is distinctly autonomous, although not radically so, the qualification being that the individual finds a sense of "completion" in another "self" and a ground of existence in that union capable of transcending all other aggregates of power. The archetypal figures that emerge in this era are personalities like Thomas More who drew from his familial ties the strength to oppose a King, and whose convictions were shaped by a belief that the nuclear family was the most potent moral, intellectual and political cell in the body politic. The marriages of the New World, cut off from kin and king alike, were exceptionally endowed with opportunity to form highly autonomous dyadic alliances. At first, theology was invoked to cultivate the new ethos; later, psychology was enlisted to rationalize its effects. The radical division of male and female roles that accompanied industrialization confirmed the "complementarity" which characterized the dyadic sense of self—a sense in which the self is "completed" by union with the "other," with one's opposite in the masculine-feminine paradigm. (Jung later refined this notion of complementary dyadic wholeness in his theory of exchanged "anima" and "animus.") Herbert Richardson describes the implications that this view holds for other relations between men and women:

> Each is regarded as incomplete in himself, and only as a man and a woman are joined sexually are they "one flesh," or one complete (androgynous) being . . . It regards sexual union as the sole possible method of becoming a complete person: a man knows himself only from sexual union with a woman and vice versa. But this is precisely why the ancient world believed that a personal, voluntary *friendship* between a man and a woman was impossible; men and women were assumed to be different kinds of beings, they could be related to each other only *sexually*, not by the moral communion of friendship—for friendship presupposes full equality and likeness of humanity in each of the persons united in this moral communion.[15]

A more radical tradition of autonomy that persisted only subliminally through both eras seems destined to emerge in our own era. The dynastic sense of self and polity dissolved long ago; today the dyadic sense is also disintegrating, chiefly because it cannot provide autonomy for both partners. We are witnessing the birth of a new age in which the individual experiences a sense of being complete in oneself. The promise of the new personality emerges out of a long tradition, both sacred and secular, of the "marginal" individual. In the ancient world, Socrates and the Sybil. Likewise, the prophets of the ancient peoples, the hermits and pilgrims, the mystics and shamans, the wandering knights, the explorers and missionaries. Jesus was an archetype in the tradition, a personality that stepped out of dynastic and dyadic self-definitions, who stripped them away from those he met, changed or healed. The type was a promise of the personality to come, the future of humanity, autonomy passing over into transcendence. The type is the archetypal solitary; and, paradoxically, the one who relates to all, who contains and at the same time transcends all.

There is a moral as well as historical prophecy contained in the words to the Galatians, which are quoted readily in our own era:

> For as many of you as were baptized into Christ have put on Christ. There is neither Jew nor Greek, there is neither slave nor free, there is neither male nor female; for you are all one in Christ Jesus.

In a political and social sense, these words contain a charter of liberation for all humanity. In a psychological and moral sense, the words suggest that Jesus unites in his personality all aspects of the human condition, as a principle of convergence that is the supreme design of the universe: "For he has made known to us in all wisdom and insight the mystery of his will according to his purpose which he set forth in Christ as a plan for the fullness of time, to unite all things in him, things in heaven and things on earth" (Ephesians 1:9). The Pauline message anticipates the coming kingdom: in the evolutionary sense that the early Church hoped for, and in the interior sense that Jesus constantly reiterated. Jesus was an archetypal androgyne, and more. He was the exemplar of solitary wholeness. Instead of a Thomas More, the boundaries of a new era are signaled by personalities such as Dag Hammarskjold, Jacques Cousteau, Mother Teresa.

In a more anthropological sense, the accelerated centripetal movements of our era may have increased the degree of pluralization and individuation in the human personality.

Teilhard de Chardin relates this phenomenon to the "convergence" at work in the cosmos. Whether it is the cells of the body or the members of a society, increased synthesis and integration—the movement toward greater unity—inevitably intensifies differentiation. As the parts of a whole blend or increase their proximity to each other, their uniqueness and incommunicability is accentuated. "The more 'other' they become in conjunction, the more they find themselves as 'self.'"[16] The "incommunicability" referred to here does not imply an absence of relationship. The solitariness of the new personality is not a separatism or narcissism (only in its demonic form). It is, rather, the solitude and aloneness that are the prerequisites of autonomy; it is a centeredness that makes union possible. Tillich distinguishes this kind of "essential solitude" from the "existential loneliness" that plagues contemporary society. Communion is possible only between persons who are rooted in this ultimate, fundamental solitude. Those who experience "loneliness" rather than "aloneness" are driven to collective involvements in which the self is sacrificed. This existential estrangement of the self dissolves the capacity for relationship into experiences of rejection, hostility, destructiveness and pain.[17] Thus, the dynastic and dyadic relationships are inevitably destructive unless they are a communion of solitudes. It would seem that the present era is a time for exploring and experimenting with new conjunctions in solitude; above all, it is a time for achieving the depth of individuation that true solitariness requires. Many of the conventional communal and conjugal structures do not promote this wholeness, largely because the "essential solitude" described by Tillich is not viewed as a necessary antecedent to those experiences.

> I wish that all were as I myself am. But each has his own special gift from God, one of one kind and one of another.
>
> To the unmarried and the widows I say that it is well for them to remain single as I do.
>
> —Paul to the Corinthians (1, 7:7–8)

Women, in particular, generally escape the necessary schooling in solitude that is crucial for autonomous, authentic relationships. Their typical life pattern transfers them from youth and family life directly into marriage and the rearing of children. Even when a space of time devoted to work intervenes, the young woman frequently lives at home or with a roommate. Living alone is a kind of existential apprenticeship that woman should require of herself for at least a part of her life-span. Unfortunately, most women are catapulted into the state of aloneness by the death of a spouse or by divorce—it is endured rather than elected.

When aloneness is consciously chosen, it is creative as well as therapeutic. The first, and perhaps most important, effect of the choice is the cultivation of an inner life. The contemporary world, with its high-speed mobility, media saturation and impersonality, tends to tribalize and robotize us at a minimal level of consciousness. We are out of touch with ourselves, with our inner feelings, with the deeper levels of experience. In proportion, our capacity for intimacy is muted. In an age that inundates us with centrifugal pulls, we need to take time to be with ourselves, centered in ourselves.

Aloneness stirs us to explore and test our own personal resources. Ways of being, doing, making and enjoying that we might never suspect ourselves capable of suddenly flower in an enlarged existential space. Like plants, people do not grow and flourish when they are crowded together. Self-esteem is enhanced by survival and coping on one's own. These life skills should be cultivated early. Young women, especially, should be coaxed out of the "herd," encouraged to pursue occasional solo experiences. Penelope Washbourn describes her own initiation into the frame of mind that transforms loneliness into autonomous expansiveness:

> I have never been very good about loneliness. When I was first in New York I didn't know many people. The men I knew in graduate school seemed not to want to date me and the girls in the dorm weren't interested in doing things I wanted to do. One day I got tired of waiting for someone to do things with and decided to go alone. So I set off into New York, myself and I went to the Metropolitan Art Museum, had lunch at a very pleasant restaurant and bought myself a ring at the museum shop . . . As the day wore on I began to experience a deep sense of pride in myself. I could have a good time alone . . . In the evening, tired after a long day I returned to the dorm. The girls asked me where I had been. "Who did you go with?" "I went alone." They could not understand it, how could anyone enjoy themselves all alone? It was a wonderful day. It put me back in touch with myself. I still have that ring, my present to myself. Whenever I feel lonely and depressed and unable to enjoy life, I look at that ring and remember my promise to myself to find joy in my aloneness.[18]

The "opening" effect that aloneness has, when deliberately chosen for its own sake, also extends to the capacity for relationship. A person whose life is not orchestrated by an exclusive and consuming commitment to one person or one family—provided, he/she is neither reclusive nor neurotic—usually shows more interest in people at large—those who are unlike oneself, unfamiliar, new on the scene, different. If fidelity is the virtue of those who are committed to each other, availability is the virtue of those who are unattached. The person who is alone must reach out, respond and construct a network of intimate relations. A sense of "belonging" and of intimacy are not "givens" for the single person—they must often be searched out or at least hoped for. Relationships are not guaranteed, they are "gifts."

This sense of person and of world as "gift" is the distinguishing element in the emergence of alternative kinship structures, networks of affiliation that are not based on the sociobiological dyad. Although these networks have existed in the past—often created out of a religious or abstract political motive—it is only in the modern era that the concept has been thoroughly secularized as a means of preserving autonomy rather than controlling it or submerging it in some higher cause (e.g., the utopian societies and religious orders). The sense of the person, the world and experience as "gift" demands a new social ideal: the ideal of a universal ecology of being, created by the transformation and/or renunciation of the limiting relationships established through biological pairing, ethnocentrism and environmental elitism.

The single life, deliberately chosen for whatever length of time, aspires to this social ideal—a solitariness that embraces the entire spectrum of human personality and experience, and at the same time, the limitations of individuality and chance. This same "openness" and unattached availability, however, give the single life a certain vulnerability to accusations of narcissism, instability, immaturity and promiscuity. As in the case of marriage, society harbors a romanticized stereotype of the single life. Unfortunately, the peer stratification and consumer culture that popularize the image of the swinging single—with everything from magazines and vacations to villages and bars for singles—help to propagate the type that it fantasizes. The public image of the single life (in advertising and the media) so often suggests that the single person is a libertine or narcissist, a spendthrift who indulges himself (herself) in frivolous pursuits, dancing, drinking, loving, loafing away the hours in the sandbox of life with the amoral innocence of a child. Unfortunately, the hustlers who have given singles a special identity are also exploiting them.

The vulnerability is real. The socialization of women, which has conditioned them to low self-esteem and a passive reactive mode of relating, has made single women particularly susceptible to the "Looking for Mr. Goodbar" syndrome. Their egos are not strong enough, self-actualized enough to choose and create an essential solitude, and so loneliness drives them to repetitive, unsatisfying and ephemeral encounters. In some women it is merely a compulsive socializing, a fear of being or doing anything alone. In its more pathological form it is masochistic and self-destructive. "Nymphomania" is a euphemism invented by males for a distinctly female phenomenon of sexual despair. One woman who has recognized herself in the "Goodbar" paradigm, describes the conflicting motives that underlie a habit of compulsive, impersonal sex: "I wanted to use men instead of having them use me; at the same time, I did it in a way that could only have been thought up by a personality already conditioned to express hostility masochistically." What is common to all of the women who act out this scenario, she observes, is that they have on a profound level, "given up hope of adequately unleashing their anger outwardly and have chosen to turn it in on themselves in a fashion that is certain to confirm their self-loathing and to win the contempt of society, too."[19]

The sexual revolution has made the single life especially problematic for women. On the one hand, the liberal woman welcomes the freedom to express her sexuality without social recrimination and restrictions. On the other, she becomes hostage to a social ethic under which "Women are not free not to be sexy." The freedom to be sexually indulgent offers little more than the opportunity to be freely exploited. Midge Decter, in proposing a new, secularized chastity, observes:

> . . . Sexual freedom has become a burden to Women's Liberation. It is burdensome not so much because of women's difficulty with the performance of its specifics as because of the larger entanglements it represents: a life in hostage to the rhythms of time and mortality, to the needs and thus the ephemerality of flesh, and to the risks of making oneself available to the demands of others.[20]

In yoking the concept of chastity to human liberation, Decter draws on a very ancient association of the idea of virginity with that of psychological autonomy and integrity. The virgin-goddess of ancient prehistory was represented as "she who is one-in-herself," but who nevertheless possessed androgynous, sexual and maternal aspects. Taylor and Diner, among others who have written about Greek and Roman society, note that the words *virgin* and *virginity* in classical literature denoted a characteristic psychological and social independence, and only when qualified with the adjective *intacta* did the terms signify biological chastity. The semantic distinction suggests an association between the idea of virginity and the achievement of an autonomous identity that cannot be realized through exclusive commitments to a husband or wife, family and children, or even through a series of successful heterosexual encounters.

The stark existential imperative contained in the ideal of chastity, epitomizes the ultimate secular vision of autonomy, as expressed by the secular conscience of Albert Camus in his *Notebooks:*

> Sex leads to nothing. It is not immoral but it is unproductive. One can indulge in it so long as one does not want to produce. But only chastity is linked to a personal progress.
>
> There is a time when sex is a victory—when it is separated from moral imperatives. But soon after it becomes a defeat—and the only victory is then won over it: chastity.[21]

The choice of this particular mode of self-fulfillment is not a denial of the importance of human relationships, however, but rather a renouncement of the emotional dependency, social compulsions and mimicry of patriarchal systems inherent in dyadic relationships. The politico-economic expediency of monogamy predisposes it to a heavy investment in permanence and exclusivity. The contemporary obsession with one-to-one, dyadic relationships is an expression, on the cultural level, of a social predicament that reveals increasing impermanence and fragmentation and, on the personal level, of an incapacity to transcend symbiotic behavior patterns that demand exclusivity.

For some women marriage does provide a maximal fulfillment of their basic needs, aspirations, and skills; it may also be instrumental in the development of personal identity and autonomy, but this cannot be guaranteed. For other women, marriage is not a satisfactory route to maximal human development, and they should choose the path of singleness with confidence and commitment. The sense of "calling" which this implies is muted, particularly in the case of women, by a social mythology that regards the single state as limbo for "left-overs." Women who avoid the bonds of matrimony and/or fulfillment in motherhood are somehow incomplete, immature even unnatural. Thus, the emancipation that the single state might bring to a woman's life is diluted by her own doubts.

Margaret Adams describes a typical example of this "deprivation" anxiety in the case of two artists, one female and one male:

In spite of obvious success, the female artist is still "ridden with disappointment" because she never married or formed a lasting relationship with a man. She is apparently not aware that this sort of involvement would interfere with her total immersion in her art; nor has she recognized that this creative impulse is the determining force in her life. Her counterpart, a male artist, the same age and also single, does not experience these same anxieties. Although his accomplishments are less than hers, he has recognized his creative potential as the overriding influence and focus of his life. He cherishes his singleness and he does not feel that he has cheated himself of experience or personal development.[22] The single woman is inhibited by several social myths which model/muddle contemporary relations between men and women:

1) *Overvalued sex.* In her survey of single men and women Margaret Adams noted that:

> Sex generally occupies a much less central place in their hierarchy of values and concerns and the practical ordering of their lives than might be expected . . . sexual enjoyment was neither rigidly rejected, zealously espoused, nor agonizingly desired; it was not regarded as the primary area of emotional investment (as it is generally credited with being), but was rather felt to be *one* facet of personal and social engagement . . .[23]

The semantic as well as cinematic nuances of a contemporary film like *An Unmarried Woman* provide some evidence of these mythic rather than realistic preoccupations. The film focuses on the compulsive efforts of a divorcée of a few weeks to pair off with almost anyone who will assuage her sexual appetite. The more critical experiences associated with divorce—property hassles and money problems, a new emphasis on one's work identity, the process of inner healing and acceptance of the finality of the separation, change of life-style, one-to-one relationships with friends, children, relatives, the sense of failure—are either conspicuously absent or downplayed in the film. Instead, the female protagonist comes off as a kind of female Don Juan, mounted securely on her newly liberated libido.

2) *Overvalued "generativity."* Erik Erikson's landmark work on the "Epigenesis of Identity" crystallized a social and psychological bias of our culture, the belief that exclusive intimate relationships are the basis of personality development. The eighth and final stage of development—"generativity"—is normally fulfilled through marriage and parenthood, or at least through the assumption of care-giving and nurturing responsibilities for the young and immature. While Erikson concedes that "some people apply this drive to other forms

of altruistic concern and creativity" it is a grudging concession, since the choice is determined "by misfortune or special and genuine gifts in other directions." As Adams points out, this attitude "keeps the nonmarriage, nonfamily style of living in the realm of the exception instead of allowing it ordinary run-of-the-mill standing . . . His approach is a subtle way of undermining the validity of the single status."[24] If Erikson's view is a temporal one, society's is not. The mythology of motherhood and the romantic dyad, and the myriad invalidations of the single life as sterile and selfish, are serious obstacles to the psychological freedom necessary to make the single life a positive choice.

There is no doubt, for example, that the acceptance in our culture of religious men and women vowed to a celibate life is at least partially explained by their traditional amalgamations in households under authority and by their dedication to works associated with nurturance and generativity. It is evident that as the traditional models give way to modern religious men and women with more independent life-styles and commitments to more worldly endeavors (law, politics, the arts), they are often subject to the same criticisms as their secular counterparts.

3) *Overpreoccupation with emulating the dyadic couple.* Compulsive heterosexual activity and "guilt" for remaining unattached negates the meaning and the essence of the single state, as we have previously noted. One of the unfortunate side effects of this overinvestment in erotic heterosexual pairing is the diminished significance of heterosexual friendship. The exclusivity which the dyadic relationship has normally implied renders an intimate friendship between a spouse or lover and someone of the opposite sex immediately suspect. The role of the friend of the opposite sex is almost unthinkable in a society in which a permanent dyadic relationship—marriage—is regarded as the fundamental basis of that society. Heterosexual friendship is too much of a threat to that exclusivity and permanence, unfortunately.

But the single person is in a unique position to override the inertial prejudice against this kind of relationship, and to explore and exploit its benefits. If everyone of the opposite sex is regarded as a potential sex partner, a person sacrifices a great deal of the privacy and integrity that makes the single life attractive, not to mention the broader spectrum of human encounters that friendship makes possible. Sociologists agree that the role of the heterosexual friend is a conspicuous and critical lacuna in our social relations. In the absence of established paradigms and scenarios for the role, the romantic-erotic dyad tends to orchestrate all one-to-one relationships. Single persons, especially, should offer conscious resistance to this emotional contamination.

The "new chastity" proposed by Midge Decter and others may help to promote the acceptance of a new mode of heterosexual friendship in our culture and inevitably benefit the married as well as the unmarried. Married persons would enjoy a wider range of interpersonal contacts and the possibility of satisfying some emotional and, perhaps, intellectual needs left unfulfilled by a spouse. The effect might be a lessening of the pressure to "be all things" to one's mate.

Perhaps the greatest challenge of the single life is the task of creating a network of relationships with persons who approve, support and perhaps share the life of radical psychological autonomy. These networks often resemble the older concept of an "extended family" and provide a sustaining nurturance, rescue potential for periods of crisis, and an opportunity for reciprocal commitment that still takes account of the basic desire to retain privacy and autonomy. These mini-systems are necessary, but often difficult to come by. Sometimes it is an accident of geographic proximity, sometimes an affinity of personal situation or common interests. More often, it is simply a question of reaching out to an available network of casual, proximate contacts who can be counted on to simply "be there." A network of friends (related or unrelated) is necessary for everyone's emotional security, but for single persons it is indispensable.

For some, a commitment to work or a way of life requires extreme rootlessness. Yet even in that rootlessness there is a certain fidelity to a kind of extended family:

> If you're a nomad—as I have been for the seventeen years I've been an actress—you find other nomads, and it becomes a giant family. You know that wherever your peculiar life leads you, you'll find a friend. There's a greatness in that, no hellos, no goodbyes. Just "catch you next time around."[25]

It is only in recent years that a few, timid apologies for the single life have begun to appear. As a way of life, the solitary existence has been conspicuously lacking in a literature that articulates the fundamental experience. Analytical insights are rare:

> Choice . . . for people who live in twos and threes and fours, is a process. Agreement is a process—a necessary self-limitation. But alone, one is the author of every choice. One's choices are one's identity, even in petty things.
>
> . . . The hardest part of living alone is exactly like the hard part of the relationship—weathering its moments of distance, its failures of insight and strength, accepting that at certain times one is powerless to affect the sadness of another—that one is sometimes powerless in the face of one's own sadness.[26]

In an era that is product-centered, task-oriented and role-dominated, the life of single autonomy represents a unique opportunity for transcendence, in both a spiritual and social sense. Thinkers have articulated the radically autonomous personality in a variety of ways: as "nomadic," as "transient," as "protean." Lifton's concept of "protean man" as a paradigm of the modern consciousness has a special relevance to the creative solitary existence. The "openness" of the deliberately chosen single life is comparable to the omniattention, polymorphous versatility, metamorphic qualities of the protean man. For protean man, as for the dedicated solitary, the capacity and opportunity for change is consciously sought. Aloneness, freedom from permanent roles becomes a "workshop of the self." Lifton, in the same vein, observes that the "image of repeated, autonomously willed death and rebirth of the self" is an image that is "very central to the protean style." Thus, it is often associated with themes of fatherlessness, family-lessness and universality. Lifton emphasizes that this protean personality is "by no means pathological," and in fact "may be one of the functional patterns necessary to life in our times."[27] Teilhard de Chardin, himself a solitary universalist, addressed this question long before Lifton's analysis, in letters dating from 1934–35:

> Why do you assume that an existence that does not succeed in taking root or bearing fruit in the form of a tangible work is less valuable than another? Why might not the World, which has need for stable families and settled poeple, need also these mobiles and wandering creatures whose action takes the form of series of seemingly unrelated trials or tests cutting across all kinds of areas?
>
> . . . We must, to a certain extent, look for a stable port, but if Life keeps tearing us away, not letting us settle anywhere, this in itself may be a call and a benediction.[28]

Lifton acknowledges the need to re-evaluate and rearticulate the whole question of stability and change, recognizing the stabilizing aspect of a dedication to change itself, as well as the possibility of change within a person whose life and role remain constant.

It is clear that in the foreseeable future, more men and significantly more women will live the single life for at least part of their life-span. Census Bureau statistics indicate that since 1970, the number of adults under thirty-five living alone has more than doubled. Among women, the rate of increase is over 120 per cent. For many it will be a necessary interlude; for others it will be a life commitment. The axiom offered by one psychiatrist, "A person who has not developed sufficient inner resources to live alone undercontributes to any relationship," suggests that singleness should at least be a prescribed apprenticeship for life, and that as a permanent lifestyle it should be lived with daring and conviction.

> Love will no longer be the intercourse of man with woman, but that of one humanity with another. And this more human love (this love full of respect and silence, sound and sure in all that it binds and looses) is indeed that for which, in strife and pain, we make ready; it consists in this, that two solitudes protect, limit and honour each other.
>
> —Rainer Maria Rilke

If there is any theme that distinguishes the fiction of Ernest Hemingway, it is the theme of love and marriage as a trap, as a web of vulnerability and self-defeat. His stories and novels, like his personal history, are saturated with a testimony of fear. Harry in *Snows of Kilimanjaro* epitomizes the fear when he says, "He could beat anything, he thought, because no thing could hurt him if he did not care." To care, to commit oneself to another, was to invite pain and loss. The major of *In Another Country* voices the same terror:

> "He cannot marry. He cannot marry," he said angrily. "If he is to lose everything, he should not place himself in a position to lose that. He should not place himself in a position to lose. He should find things he cannot lose."[29]

Hemingway choreographed his life as well as his fiction in a pattern of evasion: evasion of commitments that might lead to the pain of separation, of situations in which he could not be dominant, of relationships in which he might risk opening up his innermost self to invasion.

Ironically, it was Hemingway's fear of being alone that drove him into compulsive relationships, even after repeated failures. Unable to achieve and ground himself in essential solitude, he became a victim of existential loneliness and depression. His life is a paradigm of the fear of connectedness and the addiction to it that characteristically undermines many marriages. One who is established confidently in essential solitude, in autonomy and in the ability to take pleasure and joy in oneself as well as for oneself is one who can afford to risk connectedness and commitment.

Stanton Peele describes this as the essential difference between "love" and "addiction." The children of middle-class families are particularly susceptible to the tendency to be "addicted" to people. In a recent study, two thirds of middle-class children compared to only one fifth of lower-class children in the survey showed evidence of "social dependency constellation." The security, overprotection, lack of intimacy and materialistic focus of middle-class family life no doubt damages the child's grounding in an inner self:

> Growing up without a sense of self-assurance and self-sufficiency, we become liable to addiction in any form. And the overemphasis placed on close ties with a few individuals, together with the unavailability of other avenues for making contact with people and things causes love, marriage, and family to be the most likely objects of our addiction.[30]

Hemingway exemplifies one form of the addictive personality—emotional evasion. In the American culture, it is perhaps more characteristic of men than of women. One of Hemingway's fictional characters typifies the kind of addictive affiliation that is more common among women. Maria, in *For Whom the Bell Tolls,* wants to totally submerge herself in her lover, at the expense of her own identity: "I would be thee because I love thee so." Jordan's reply is rather atypical for Hemingway: "It is better to be one and each one to be the one he is."

Women, more than men, are victimized by addictive socialization. They are generally more brainwashed by the notion that "you can't make it alone," by the idea that survival is dependent upon an exclusive attachment, or upon what Gail Sheehy describes as "merging." Low self-esteem, insufficient experience in coping with her own resources and creating the circumstances of her own life, and economic and biological contingency are all factors that contribute to emotional dependency and addiction in many women:

> The role mapped out for a woman symbolizes the addict's lot because it is predicated on inadequacy. A woman is expected to be an empty, formless vessel, shaped by whoever or whatever comes along to fill her up. Any activity undertaken out of this lack of personal completeness is likely to become an addiction. Conventionally, women have been channeled into a few basic involvements—marriage, family, home. These personal relationships constitute women's assigned sphere of activity. It is not surprising if, lacking other outlets, a woman defines herself by such relationships and depends on them to the point of addiction.[31]

If, indeed, "the test of our secure being, of our connectedness is the capacity to enjoy being alone," why would anyone marry at all?

The Hemingway evasion, maneuvering oneself into a position of safety, where one "cannot lose," is a kind of death wish. It is the same misdirected notion of freedom that recurs so frequently in contemporary popular music, reminiscent of the line from the Kristofferson-Foster song that goes, "Freedom's just another word for nothing left to lose." The immunity and complacency implied in this notion of freedom are life-and-growth-denying instincts. Likewise, the compulsive need to bury one's identity in another person. The decision to love, to marry, to raise a family, to be committed to something or someone and still retain one's autonomy—is a decision to risk everything. But risking everything is the highest expression of autonomy, of personal freedom. Freud recognized this when he observed, "Life is impoverished, it loses in interest, when the highest stake in living, life itself, may not be risked."

The mystery of marriage, of unconditional commitment, is much the same as the mystery at the heart of the great religions of humanity—the mystery of total self-sufficiency, the Absolute Being, sharing itself, containing its limitless energy in diminished form, communicating itself by calling forth being in new forms. To love is to place oneself—all that one is—in a position to be "called forth" to new dimensions, to expressions of being. As we do not achieve consciousness unless someone converses with us—calls us to greater being—in infancy, so at any stage of life, encounter with and commitment to others brings us to a threshold of new consciousness, of greater being, of growth. Self-making is a process of continuous communion. It is fraught with challenge and pain. Those who immunize their autonomy by evading love, or those who anesthetize their autonomy by immersing it in another identity, remain infants in the spiritual sense—they cannot create themselves by continually transcending themselves. They never reach the maturity of theonomy.

Paradoxically, the risk of theonomous love depends on a high degree of self-confidence and self-sufficiency, and at the same time on a recognition of the uncertainty and contingency of a relationship that ultimately transcends one's own control and will. This gives the creative relationship a dynamic and dialectical quality; conviction and doubt marry each other. As Rollo May puts it: "We must be fully committed, but we must also be aware at the same time that we might possibly be wrong."[32] This dialectic is of the essence of the creative love commitment and its greatest insurance against stagnation and self-deception.

Again, one might seek out love and commitment on one's own terms. Why bother to marry?

For most people, marriage is like skiing. In the beginning one is propelled from the precipice by "love" or necessity, by reasons that in themselves are inadequate to sustain the project that has been undertaken. One finds oneself speeding down a slope—to go back is impossible; to stop might be catastrophic. The momentum, combined with unexpected hazards and turns and an uncertain end, create an overwhelming concentration and tension. The sense of risk, particularly for the inexperienced, is both exhilarating and terrifying. So often there is no time or no space for evaluating just what has been risked. Love "happens"; one finds oneself married before one has evaluated the stakes. The game commences before we know the rules. Margaret Atwood provides a particularly illuminating scenario of the marriage question in her novel *Surfacing*. The heroine has caught herself in the vertigo of descent:

> "How do you manage it?" I said.
>
> She stopped humming. "Manage what?"
>
> "Being married. How do you keep it together?"
>
> She glanced at me quickly as though she was suspicious.

> "We tell a lot of jokes."
>
> "No, but really," I said. If there was a secret trick I wanted to learn it.
>
> She talked to me then, or not to me exactly but to an invisible microphone suspended above her head: people's voices go radio when they give advice. She said you just had to make an emotional commitment, it was like skiing, you couldn't see in advance what would happen, but you had to let go. Let go of what I wanted to ask her; I was measuring myself against what she was saying. Maybe that was why I failed, because I didn't know what I had to let go of. For me it hadn't been like skiing, it was more like jumping off a cliff. That was the feeling I had all the time I was married; in the air, going down, waiting for the smash at the bottom.[33]

The heroine seems to sense that she has sacrificed something she shouldn't have—her autonomy. The risks of marriage should be those of maintaining autonomy, of living tandem in spite of different rates of growth, unexpected crises and mutual mistakes. It should not mean the invalidation of the self, the loss of essential solitude.

Later in the novel the heroine compares marriage to a game of Monopoly or a crossword puzzle. In this analogy with the structure of games and the human instinct to "play" perhaps lies the ultimate rationale for conventional marriage. Play is the symbolic representation of the human capacity for "risk," and at the same time, of the human passion for order. Playing fields, playgrounds and game tables are consecrated spots, hedged around and hallowed, within which special rules obtain. All are temporary worlds within the ordinary world. All involve risk and hazard, rules and penalties, and the exigencies of chance and the unexpected. All bring participants into intense confrontation and intimacy, and the feeling of being apart together in an exceptional situation, of sharing something important. Into an imperfect world and into the confusion of life it brings a temporary, limited experience of order and coherence, from which meaning emerges.

The instinct to marry (to distinguish it from the impulse to love) is an analogous one. The elements proper to play are also indigenous to marriage: order, tension, movement, change, seriousness, rhythm, rapture, release. Above all, it is a reflection of the need to give meaning and form to life. Marriage has an aesthetic basis similar to the principle of limitation in art: The stricter the form, the more perfect the art. Marriage, as an unconditional commitment, imposes the limitations that make a creative relationship possible, just as form provides the essential boundaries and structure for the creative act. As a form, it springs from the unconscious as well as from the conscious perception of custom. (The "triadic" form recurs in dreams, suggesting not only the primordial familial structure but also the dialectic of self with "other" and the inner dialectic which is a synthesis of it.)

The married insert themselves deliberately in the time frame of history and enjoy the sense of continuity and coherence that this conveys. "In marrying, we pick up our destinies in a large album of kinship and family. It is this sense of jumping into a time frame of place and connections that distinguishes marriage from other forms of living arrangements."[34] The married step into the precise confines of a photograph or painting—the frame gives it a certain meaning. The unmarried must chisel the form and meaning of their lives out of a comparatively undifferentiated block of marble—matter and space are more subject to their manipulation. Thus, marriage often represents a commitment to an existing value system, whereas the unmarried are free to forge a relationship model that echoes or subverts conventional value systems or to create new ones undreamed of.

For married and unmarried alike, however, the album of kinship and family must be exorcised. Stepping into the time frame of marriage is so often like stepping into the carnival photographer's tent: We don an old-fashioned costume from the trunkful supplied, and we sit for a "family" portrait in front of an old-fashioned camera. In the finished photo, we look more like our ancestors than like ourselves. We play the parts with unconscious aplomb. If our own relationships are to be free and creative, we must divest ourselves of some of these masks, costumes and scripts that linger, ready-to-wear, in the attic of the soul.

One of the most hermetic of Jesus' sayings in the New Testament is recorded in Matthew 10:34–35, "I have come to set a man against his father, and a daughter against her mother, and a daughter-in-law against her mother-in-law," and in Luke 14:26, "If anyone comes to me and does not hate his own father and mother and wife and children and brothers and sisters, yes, and even his own life, he cannot be my disciple." As a message of transcendence, the prophetic words seem to imply a calling forth beyond the security of the conventional familial structures. The personal meaning of these words, at least in a psychological sense, has perhaps been articulated best by the contemporary anti-psychiatrists. Cooper, for example, says,

> One has to see through one's family into the inviting but somewhat murky world of other people outside it . . . Before one arrives at any marital relationship with other people in the world outside one's family, one has to go through a whole lot of divorce proceedings with each of these people to a more or less partial or total degree. One may finally have to get divorced from one's relationship with one of one's parents, or divorced from one's infatuation with their marriage, and so on, seriatim, through the sibling ranks and the ranks of "significant others."[35]

This kind of emotional divorce is necessitated by what R. D. Laing calls the "fantasy of the family"—an introjected set of relations learned in the family, which are subsequently "mapped" onto other relationships.[36] Each person's identity rests on a shared "family imago" inside the other members of the family. This family set of relations becomes a set of tapes, of scenarios structuring all of one's actions; it can be mapped onto every aspect of the cosmos, onto the entire spectrum of relationships, groups and institutions. This transference must be eliminated if we are to connect with others in authentic, free and autonomous relations. The phenomenon has a spectral aspect, in that one generation becomes a kind of psychic burial plot of the preceding one:

> We induce others, and are ourselves induced, to *embody* them: to enact, unbeknown to ourselves, a shadow play, as images of images of images . . . of the dead, who have in their return embodied and enacted such dreams projected upon them, and induced in them, by those before them . . .
>
> We are acting parts in a play that we have never read and never seen, whose plot we don't know, whose existence we can glimpse, but whose beginning and end are beyond our present imagination and conception . . .
>
> Until one can see the "family" in oneself one can see neither oneself nor any family clearly . . .
>
> If I do not destroy the "family," the "family" will destroy me.[37]

The dilemma of Goldilocks, aspiring to self-actualization in relationship, but confronted with ill-fitting roles, can be resolved only by conscious exorcism. Marriages constellated according to unauthentic patterns serve neither partner. Many of these patterns and scenarios are buried in the semantic deep structure of the basic pledge of the marriage compact: "I love you." Translated, it might mean—as it does for many women—"There are things about you that I don't like or shouldn't tolerate—but *I'll reform you*" (the patriarchal role of moral dominance) or, "I am a warm, loving, giving person, *I'll meet all of your needs*" (the maternal role of total nurturance) or, "I'll be and do anything you want, in return for your love" (the subservient, plastic "child" role).

Lest one's family of origin be blamed for too much pathology, another source of affiliation modeling should be recognized—the peer group. Especially since the 1960s, peer-bonding has been viewed as the ideal model for an egalitarian relationship. Essentially a twinship of amoral and irresponsible immaturity, it often masquerades as a union of autonomous equals or "playmates": "The idealized comradeship of siblings, united not by undying passion or even mutual respect but merely by a common resentment of adult authority, becomes the model of the perfect marriage."[38] Exorcism is complete, one is ready for authentic relationship only when, to paraphrase Dostoyevsky, one assumes total responsibility *for* oneself, *to* one's partner, and *for* everything. The heroine of the novel *Surfacing* successfully demythologizes her "family fantasy," and emerges from a voyage to the edge of madness, cleansed and confident, the husks of old relationships shed forever:

> No total salvation, resurrection, Our father, Our mother I pray, Reach down for me, but it won't work: they dwindle, grow, become what they were, human. Something I never gave them credit for; but their totalitarian innocence was my own . . .
>
> This above all, to refuse to be a victim. Unless I can do that I can do nothing. I have to recant, give up the old belief that I am powerless and because of it nothing I can do will ever hurt anyone . . .
>
> . . . We can no longer live in spurious peace by avoiding each other, the way it was before, we will have to begin. For it's necessary, the intercession of words; and we will probably fail, sooner or later, more or less painfully. That's normal, it's the way it hap-

> pens now and I don't know whether it's worth it or even if I can depend on him, he may have been sent as a trick. But he isn't an American, I can see that now; he isn't anything, he is only half formed, and for that reason I can trust him.
>
> To trust is to let go . . .[39]

The risk of marriage makes sense only when both partners have preserved their autonomy, are unencumbered by old scripts and scenarios, and are totally open to the future of each other.

> She was not at all sure that it was this mutual unison in separateness that she wanted . . . she knew he would never abandon himself finally to her. He did not believe in final self-abandonment. He said it openly. It was his challenge. She was prepared to fight him for it. For she believed in an absolute surrender to love. She believed that love far surpassed the individual. He said that the individual was *more* than love, or than any relationship. For him, the bright, single soul accepted love as one of its conditions, a condition of its own equilibrium.
>
> —D. H. Lawrence, *Women in Love*

Much of the current disillusionment with marriage among women is a perception of its failure to be what it promises: a creative partnership. Residual role stereotypes and social structures frustrate the sharing of work, homemaking and child rearing that true partnership demands. Moreover, after the first decade, stagnation often sets in. A relationship that should have nurtured personal growth and creativity begins to have the opposite effect. Far too much was expected of an exclusive relationship; other nutrients that might have been cultivated outside the marriage dry up, the couple isolate themselves on the desert island of suburbia, and it is no paradise. The call of Genesis to "increase and multiply" is sterilized in the most significant and spiritual dimension which the words imply.

The dyadic qualities of the traditional marriage will not sustain the "new" women. The fundamental structure of the relationship must change. Two elements in particular will diminish in the "new" marriages: *complementariness* (in terms of psychological needs and conjugal roles) and *exclusivity* (in the broader sense of the scope of friends, networks, and involvement beyond the couple). As with sex, we have reduced marriage in the dyadic mode to an obsession with moments of *orgasmic togetherness.* The fantasy of complete self-transcendence in a relationship, like the fantasy of the ultimate, perfect orgasm, is fundamentally a death fantasy. If the new "eco-self" is to survive and flourish in a marriage compact, the marriage itself must become an expansive and inclusive ecosystem.

This systemic expansion arises from the increased intensity of interpersonal relations as well as the impacted, centripetal quality of contemporary life. "Crowded more and more together, we are learning to live more distantly from one another, in strategically varied and numerous contacts, rather than in the oppressive warmth of family and a few friends."[40] More private space, more time for each partner to be a "self." Silence, absence. The fortress of the traditional dyad must give way to an open-air canopy. This openness, however, need not mean total availability. Priority should be placed on those things the married couple enjoy in common, shared worlds beyond the intimacies of the bedroom and the tasks of making a home. The greater the range of shared interests beyond the requirement of conjugal living, the better. There should also be other things—friends, jobs, pursuits—which they do not have in common. The precise combination, the "magic mix" will be a constant challenge. This expansion of the conjugal system to include many more relational networks obviously will require a major reordering of time and work priorities. In order to broaden the base of the family and share more in a qualitative sense, a couple may have to elect a lower standard of living in preferring a less time-consuming or stress-inducing kind of work. Because the conjugal system is more open and the persons more multi-faceted, more choices will have to be made, and more communication will be necessary to sustain the equilibrium. But the very act of continually confronting it as a process, and as an evolving vision, gives the relationship momentum. Conjugal soul-making is choreographic, and over the years it creates that sense of a "shared sacred history" that is, finally, the ultimate reason for staying together. The permanence of the marriage bond is its fruit, not its root.

If the partners are sufficiently protean and unselfish, they may indeed construct a permanent relationship in which all of the possible ends of marriage are fulfilled, at least sequentially. The broadened base of the marriage, while it presents many challenges may also increase the chances for a long-term survival of the relationship. For many men and women, however, the probability that any one spouse or any one marriage will meet their life-long needs and aspirations is decreasing. Anthropologists have described the emergence of a new pattern in our culture, the "three-marriage" life cycle: a first, youthful marriage for romance; a second for the establishment of a family; a third, in later years, for companionship. Each of these relationships is qualitatively distinct, and each usually corresponds to a particular stage or plateau in psychological development. Growth away from one stage toward the next is inevitable—if two people cannot accomplish this in concert, they may have to dissolve the relationship. One partner may skip a stage or remain fixated at one level.

We expect all of our relationships, like all of our fairy tales, to end "happily ever after." Most of them end, as life itself does, in some kind of separation and loss, in a mini-death. Divorce, the most catastrophic of these experiences, can be a breakthrough experience, a death and dying process that leaves us changed. One woman describes this process:

> The end of my marriage shattered my growing sense of complacency and pride at my own success. I was unmasked and that prideful girl was no more. Gradually, from the silence of the months of pain I began to talk to friends that I had cut off from seeing my anguish. At first I heard only my self-pity as I told the story of the failure of my hope. Gradually, the immediate grief faded and I began to build. I started to recognize my own complicity in our failure to risk or to trust communication. I discovered old and new friendships and the ability to learn trust again. The divorce aged me, it stripped me bare of my false pretenses of innocence and self-satisfaction. I recognized unconscious drives and motivations in myself as the result of the failure of that marriage. Maybe nothing has been more productive of growth in myself than what I initially experienced as a death.[41]

For most women, in spite of the redeeming insights that it may bring, divorce is a shattering experience fraught with pain, anguish and enmity. If it frees one from bondage and victimization, it also leaves one with permanent scars and guilts. If there is relief and respite, there is also abandonment and estrangement—loss of some friends, confusion of children, dismay of relatives, loneliness, economic and social jeopardy. Above all, it is the sense of failure and self-doubt that is perhaps the most terrifying and debilitating effect of divorce.

In a curious way, it is also the sense of failure that may be the cause, not merely the result of divorce. The "death of love," in fact, may be a suicide. The alarming increase of suicides among college students and teenagers has been directly allied to feelings of failure, of inability to cope with expectations projected by parents and peers. Fear of failure to achieve a life-task ambition, like fear of failure in a life task itself, generates self-destructive gestures and feelings of despair. Socialization in our society has apparently not taught young people how to distinguish psychologically between failure at a task and failure as a person. The two are often confused in the minds of the young, and the pressure to achieve in the face of diminishing possibilities can devastate their fragile egos. They give up rather than adapt, reconstruct or redesign their lives.

The marriage bond exhibits many analogous stresses and responses. In a society characterized by change, insecurity and a high degree of mobility, the marriage pair-bond becomes more critical. As kinship, neighborhood and institutional relational structures dissolve, interpersonal relations become freighted with added significance. Our expectations of marriage are probably the highest in the history of civilization. Our disillusionment, when these expectations are not met, is equally profound. Thus, the projection of failure—personal and mutual—is undoubtedly one of the most crucial internal factors affecting the durability of marriages in our society today. The best proof of the exaggerated expectations Americans harbor concerning marriage is the high rate of remarriage. Census data from 1970 shows that five out of six divorced men and three out of four divorced women remarry:

> Despite a high legal divorce rate, a high proportion is married—higher than in any other industrial society. Americans expect a great deal out of the state of wedlock, and when a particular marriage proves unsatisfactory, they seek to dissolve it and try again.[42]

As with automobiles, Americans abhor "obsolescence" in relationships—they would rather replace something than attempt to repair or rebuild it. Divorce is sometimes the easy way out, particularly when the marriage has been undermined by self-distrust and failed expectations. There is a utopian element in this American attitude toward marriage, and when the reality fails to live up to the fantasy, the experiment is frequently abandoned.

Christian marriage offers at the same time the most idealistic and most realistic paradigm for marriage. On one level it risks the ultimate. It deliberately promises what in fact it cannot deliver—fidelity, permanence. In doing this, however, it introduces a third "presence" into the compact of the married couple—a promise that has the power to summon the man and woman over and over again to a new existence, a new being. The relationship itself is thus a presence emanating from the pledge, which constantly demands and motivates transcendence; the pledge is itself a cause and the means to fidelity. The pledge makes it possible for consent to be born again in the face of change and novelty. It is not rigid adherence to a prior decision or principle, but the unchanging gift of oneself to a loved one.

Truly this is folly, some will say. How can one have adequate grounds, adequate knowledge of self to make a permanent gift of oneself? Gabriel Marcel and some of the existentialists seem to offer a better answer to this question than Descartes: "In principle, to commit myself I must first know myself; the fact is, however, that I really know myself only when I have committed myself."[43] How do I know where to go except by going?

On another level, Christian marriage provides a realistic scheme for marriage. It is assumed that both partners are likely to err, to disappoint one another—but the Christian compact also provides a structure of belief, of forgiveness and healing of memory, to sustain the married couple. The lovers alone will decide the parameters of this mutual amnesty. These moments of reconciliation, like the initial pledge of lasting fidelity, transcend what either partner might be capable of without a belief structure—they become moments of grace. They can be, and often are, moments of growth, new beginnings. All men and women, however, are capable of being selfish and stupid, lazy and aggressive, bitter and treacherous. They can exploit, manipulate and harm one another. They can fail to evangelize their marriage; one or the other partner can become an insurmountable obstacle to the human development and spiritual growth of the other. Christian marriages have mortal limits, and often divorce is a final act of caring when all else has failed.

It is ironic that the teaching of the Catholic Church concerning divorce should be so devoid of this element, when in fact it was

Jesus "caring" for the situation of women in his day that provoked his words concerning the indissolubility of marriage.

> He did not hesitate to challenge the Deuteronomic law on divorce, which was entirely male-oriented (Deut. 24:1–4) in the name of the earlier myth of creation. By quoting Genesis 2:23–24, Jesus made it clear that he understood the reality of the mutual responsibility and the obligation of love between a husband and a wife (Matt. 19:3ff.). It is ironical to observe, however, that his insistence on the indissolubility of marriage, which represented an attempt to support defenseless women, has become the ground for a new form of legalism.[44]

We live in a society that is moving inexorably toward a norm of consecutive plural marriage. Divorce can no longer be regarded solely as a consequence of personal rigidities and inability to adjust, or of spiritual reprobation. We must recognize it as a potentially creative rather than destructive act, a valid, moral, sanctioned social invention, an orderly instrument of change.

Christians, perhaps, can go a step farther in "caring." Some churches have instituted a ceremony of reconciliation for divorcing partners. Sometimes the process of religious preparation for divorce provides a "discernment" experience that leads to a reunion. When it does not, the couple must be helped to part in compassion, in a state of self-realization rather than self-destruction.

> The religious community celebrates and commemorates, through symbol and ceremony, the most significant events in the maturation cycle: birth, marriage, and finally death. There are even rites for such important occasions as serious illness, school graduation or moving into a new home. Why not, then, recognize liturgically the crucial impact of the divorce experience? Even today, for all of the supposed sophistication toward the subject of divorce, two persons in the process of divorce will need the support of their friends and religious community almost more than they will at any other time in their lives.[45]

The insertion of divorce into a religious dimension is a recognition that although a legal commitment may be dissolved, a relationship is changed but not ended. In Robert Anderson's *I Never Sang for My Father,* the final lines of the play are a profound testimony to the transcendence that is the essence of a relationship. The bereaved son says, "Death ends a life, but it does not end a relationship which struggles on in the survivor's mind toward some resolution which it never finds . . ." Divorce ends a marriage, but not a relationship. And survival is a soul-making experience.

We were Siamese twins.
Our blood's not sure
if it can circulate,
now we are cut apart.
Something in each of us is waiting
to see if we can survive,
severed.

—Denise Levertov, "Divorcing"

Each of us sets out in search of a "perfect family," one that mirrors the image we carry around inside of us, one that will nurture and support us, one that we ourselves can create and mold, one that we feel comfortable in, one that will stretch our being to its full height.

These relationships are constantly shifting, like stars in the night sky. We no sooner test the limits of one than we are launched into another, into a new constellation.

We are always the stranger, the intruder. We are the golden-haired innocent or the cunning fox. We are the dancer encircling the dance. We fly from things become to things becoming. We bring nothing to these encounters unless we bring our own solitude. The forest is before, and it is after.

One is potency, readiness and presence (it can also be abdication).

Two is security, affirmation and care-fulness (it can also be incest).

Is it not *three* that we hope for and make ready for?

> Suddenly it happened. The encounter became a family, passion a work of love. Torment and fear turned into rules and pacts. The theme changed from fire to a piece to be forged, to an object to be situated. Encirclement, a circle, a parabola. An open parabola.
>
> Once hesitant sisters, each of us adorning ourselves in our own feathers, one of you in lyrical, emotional outpourings and erot-

icism, the other of you in "analytical distance," and I in ironic detachment, each of us the prisoner of her pretended strength, in the heat of what was happening, we found ourselves touched by, revealed in the common childhood that we made it our task to discover, sharing our grievances with each other, and in so doing gaining the courage to accuse and suspect each other, going on from accusing our mothers to accusing each other to our faces, and discovering that we could tolerate this—and that is how we made each of ourselves the mother and the daughter of each of the others, and sisters determined to talk about precisely why we were orphans and suffering and destitute. A new family.

All this linked in a chain, each of us intermingling and trying on forms of the others, as though attempting to possess each other, and succeeding in so doing, each of us impregnating first one and then the other of the two in turn.

. . . This is not the house of pairs. Poor, poor couples who are only two! Three is the end of virginity, the beginning of the true history of equal partners. (*The Three Marias: New Portuguese Letters*[46])

the legend

The story's essence is not just the growth of Beauty's love for the Beast, or even her transferring her love for her father to the Beast, but her own growth in the process. From believing that she must choose between her love for her father and her love for the Beast, Beauty moves to the happy discovery that seeing these two loves in opposition is an immature view of things . . .

The marriage of Beauty to the former Beast is a symbolic expression of the healing of the pernicious break between the animal and the higher aspects of man—a separation which is described as a sickness, since, when separated from Beauty and what she symbolizes, first her father and then the Beast nearly die.

—Bruno Bettelheim, *The Uses of Enchantment*[1]

Yet now that she had come face to face with it, the Minotaur resembled someone she knew. It was not a monster. It was a reflection upon a mirror, a masked woman, Lillian herself, the hidden masked part of herself unknown to her, who had ruled her acts. She extended her hand toward this tyrant who could no longer harm her. It lay upon the mirror of the plane's round portholes, traveling through the clouds, a fleeting face, her own, clear and definable only when darkness came.

—Anaïs Nin, *Seduction of the Minotaur*[2]

In the light of her new consciousness she experiences a fateful transformation, in which she dis-

covers that the separation between beast and husband is not valid. As the lightning bolt of love strikes her, she turns the knife against her own heart or (in other terms) wounds herself on Eros' arrow. With this she departs from the childlike, unconscious aspect as well. Only in a squalid, lightless existence can Psyche mistake her lover for a beast, a violator, a dragon, and only as a childishly ignorant girl (but this too is a dark aspect) can she suppose that she is in love with a "higher husband" distinct from the lower dragon. In the light of irrupting love Psyche recognizes Eros as a god, who is the upper and the lower in one, and who connects the two . . .

With Psyche's love that burst forth when she "sees Eros," there comes into being within her an Eros who is no longer identical with the sleeping Eros outside her. This inner Eros that is the image of her love is in truth a higher and invisible form of the Eros who lies sleeping before her.

—Erich Neumann, *Amor and Psyche*[3]

All fairy tales are about transformation, metamorphosis. There are two recurring variations on the theme: One, in which the heroine's situation is suddenly, dramatically and instantly changed for the better—usually by some extrinsic intervention. The other, in which the change or revelation takes place after a long, arduous struggle and is the result of the heroine's own growth in self-knowledge and moral capacity. *Beauty and the Beast* belongs to this latter kind; almost every language and culture has a tale based on its theme. It has supplied us with more variations in stories, poems, novels, plays, film and dance than perhaps any other fairy tale. More than any other tale, it celebrates self-knowledge and self-transcendence. It is about love as a principle of deification, or as Chesterton put it, about the truth that "a thing must be loved before it is loveable."

Beauty and the Beast, and its numerous derivatives in the "animal bridegroom" genre, are descended from a more ancient archetypal myth—the story of Cupid (Eros) and Psyche. Abandoned to a marriage with a "monster" (who is really the god Eros), Psyche is forbidden to look on her divine consort and they meet as lovers only in the darkness of night. Seduced by her sisters, she disobeys the injunction of her husband-god and looks upon him with a lamp while he sleeps. He awakens, wounded by the oil from her lamp, and abandons her. Psyche pines for his return and undergoes a series of arduous tasks. In one of her ordeals she even descends to the underworld. Finally, Eros returns to her, his wound healed with the balm of her remorse. To placate his mother, Aphrodite, he asks Zeus to confer the immortality of the gods on Psyche, and Psyche is "caught up" into the heavens for her divine nuptials. Erich Neumann suggests the evolutionary and transcendent significance of this myth:

> Through her ascension to Olympus she demonstrates that a new epoch has begun. That Psyche has become a goddess means that the human is itself divine and equal to the gods; and the eternal union of the goddess Psyche with the god Eros means that the human bond with the divine is not only eternal, but itself of a divine quality.
>
> Strangely enough, the tale of Psyche thus represents a development which in an extra-Christian era, without revelation and without church, wholly pagan and yet transcending paganism, symbolizes the transformation and deification of the psyche.[4]

A crucial aspect of the myth is thus Psyche's self-actualizing creative power—she performs a decisive act while Eros sleeps, then endures the consequences. Her loss does not immobilize her, but engages her in an unrelenting search for Eros, and a willingness to bear many trials. Psyche—the archetype of the soul—progresses from heteronomy to autonomy, and finally to redemptive theonomy. The union of Eros and Psyche symbolizes the integration of transcendence and immanence, divine power manifested in human wisdom.

The Beast emerges from the human imagination as a projection of its own alienation from itself and from the ground of its being, which is God. Like Eros, what is suppressed, unacknowledged, misunderstood is first projected as monstrous, as radically Other. When Beauty offers herself as ransom for her father, she accepts a transcendent summons to greater being. Her name, "Beauty," contains a promise of beatitude, which she will be worthy of because she has preferred virtue to pleasure and wealth. In Madame Leprince de Beaumont's version of the tale, the best-known modern variant, Beauty accepts the poverty of her father's financial collapse and the servitude it necessitates—she humbles herself among her siblings, and is therefore more beloved of her father. Her attentiveness to the inner life is suggested in the contrasts that are drawn between her and her sisters: "They spent their time promenading about, going to balls and plays, and looked down on their young sister who spent most of her time reading at home."

The father's theft of a rose from the Beast's garden and his gift of it to his innocent daughter, along with the punishment that will be exacted for it, is a kind of parable of the transmission of original sin. Because she is innocent and virtuous, she alone can redeem her family from their fallen state. So, in spite of her fear of being devoured, Beauty chooses to become the Beast's prisoner.

She gradually discovers, to her surprise, that she is master in the Beast's castle: "Desire, command. Here, you are the Queen; you are the mistress." In allowing her to return to visit her father the Beast gives her ultimate power over himself. In Jean Cocteau's film version of the tale,[5] the empowerment is even more emphatic when the Beast gives her the key to Diana's lodge as a pledge of his trust in her: "It is the only place on the estate that no one may enter, nor you, nor I. All I possess, I possess by magic, but my true wealth is in this lodge."

When Beauty returns home, she finds more evidence of the uniqueness of the power she has received. When she tries to give away the gifts which the Beast has given her, the jewelry is transformed—the pearl necklace is metamorphosed into a strand of burned rope. Her father cautions her: "What the Beast has offered you is yours. You can't give it to anyone else."

What Beauty has received and cannot give away, without dire consequences for everyone, is her own personal autonomy and empowerment. Beauty has come into possession of herself; and in coming to love herself, the fear of the "Other" dissolves, the Beast becomes a friend. The theme of self-knowledge, identity and autonomy is illuminated even more in the recent Hallmark Hall of Fame production of the fairy tale. When she inquires whether she might learn more about the Beast from the books in her room, he tells her that the books have been left there so she may learn more about *herself*. The process of self-discovery is underscored by her own admissions: "If I do discover that I love you, I must hate myself," and then, "I like your touch, I loathe myself for liking it."

As Beauty discovers the "beast" in herself, she discovers the god in the Beast. In her betrayal, she recognizes her own complicity in evil and transcends it with an act of love: "I'm the one that is the monster, my Beast." Because she has accepted the Beast in the truth of his ugliness, without the illusion of sentiment (in the Hallmark version, he has the face of a pig), and because she has seen into her own darkness of soul, the "Otherness" of the Beast dissolves, the spell is broken.

Beauty and the Beast is a symbolic representation of a soul in the process of exorcising patriarchal images—benevolent as well as threatening—that wield power over it. There are no mothers in this fable—only fathers, who are the source of the domestic, social and religious dependence of women. But the process of liberation is seen to be two-sided: The *objective situation* can only be modified by first changing the *subjective consciousness.* The dualism of Beauty and Beast must be dissolved before the dream of wholeness and oneness can be realized.

Another cycle of tales, the "forbidden chamber" genre, presents a variation on the *Beauty and the Beast* theme. *"Bluebeard"* is perhaps the best-known version today; it tells of a woman who, married to a "monster," disobeys her husband's express prohibition during his absence, and opens a certain door, behind which she finds the mutilated corpses of her predecessors. Her disobedience is discovered by the husband from a telltale bloodstain upon the key, and he is about to add her to his morbid collection in the "forbidden chamber" when he is killed by her rescuing brothers or friends. In one group of these tales the husband is the Devil, and the forbidden door closes the entrance to Hell.

In this tale, the woman's invasion into the man's hidden chamber is a breach of patriarchal etiquette: "The female must not inquire into the secrets of the male." As Bettelheim observes, these proscriptions concerning the hidden chamber are always a test of a wife's faithfulness to her husband's authority. When the wife's curiosity (autonomy) overpowers her sense of subservience, she discovers the truth—that rather than allow any woman to have an existence apart from himself, her spouse would rather kill her. There is no wisdom, kindness, or courtesy in Bluebeard as there is in the Beast.

The heroine of this tale cannot achieve a rapprochement—she cannot act autonomously. Her weakness requires intervention by others who will rescue her. (With a few possible exceptions: notably, a Gaelic and a Basque version of the tale in which *she* kills the monster-husband!)

Moreover, in the resolution of the story, neither she nor her partner is transformed. Transcendence is impossible; destruction is the only alternative. Neither the objective situation nor the subjective consciousness can be modified. Hence, the situation must simply be *dissolved, escaped* and *denied.* Thus, in Perrault's version, the heroine finally seeks marriage "with a very worthy man, who banished from her mind all memory of the evil days she had spent with Bluebeard."

These two tales deal symbolically with the incarceration of women in a psychological as well as sociopolitical sense. The patriarchy is within as well as without. Shall the Beast/Bluebeard be exorcised or executed? Can the past be redeemed, or must it be rejected? Can God be reborn?

Beauty is one of the few fairy-tale heroines that we think of as having reached maturity before the story begins. She is in command of herself, she lives in harmonious relationship with her inner world as well as with her surroundings, she is happy. Her father's mistake intrudes on her peace of soul, presents a dilemma that can be solved only by her act of sacrifice. When she gives herself up as ransom for her erring father, it is not a compulsive act, a masochistic reflex or the result of her devaluation of herself. She freely modifies her autonomy in the interests of a higher good. She confronts the Beast in her life, symbolic not only of what she has hidden in her own psyche, but of all those "close encounters" with alien, threatening life experiences, all the passivities and diminishments—unanticipated and unmerited—that rupture human happiness. She enters willingly into a dark night of the soul, experiencing fright, confusion and frustration. She looks on the face of a fierce God. By confronting and accepting it, she transforms it into her own likeness, until finally the spell is broken, the beloved one is released and revealed, the kingdom renewed.

FIVE

Beauty Exorcises the Beast

HISTORIANS and sages are fond of attributing the improved status of women in the Western world to everything from Christianity and democracy to the printing press. But every modern woman knows in her heart that her real liberation began with the Pill. Flawed as it is, and full of hazard, the Pill is more than a chemical contraceptive. It is a symbol of the new technological, psychological and social power of woman over her own biology—and ultimately over her own life.

The Pill is a metaphor for the contemporary woman's discovery of autonomy. In assuming more independent control over her own body, the "new woman" declared her right to control her own time, life span, life-style and self-image. She was no longer hostage to the implacable forces of fertility, social mythology and dogmatism. She need no longer be sacrificed to the unknown gods of "nature," no longer driven to self-mutilations in defending the integrity of her life. She began to experience a wider spectrum of options, the kind men have always taken for granted. She began to choose, and thus to grow.

Her body became a new source of self-esteem and creative energy. The misogynist disgust for female anatomy (which women have always absorbed, like blotters, from their milieu) was dissolved in the transformation of her sexuality from something apart from herself into a wholistic expression of her essential being—no longer an object, but an agent of existence. Vaginal pride replaced penis envy, confirming Nancy Friday's maxim, "Convince a woman that her vagina is beautiful, and you have the makings of an 'equal' person."[6]

The empowerment of women in the twentieth century coincided with the rising aspirations of subjugated races and disenfranchised minorities on a worldwide scale. For women, the possibility of control over their bodies—their lives—is analogous to the economic and political empowerment of underdeveloped peoples. And the two are inextricably intertwined, as many revolutionary struggles currently attest.

But the assumption of autonomy—whether personal or political—is not an unqualified transformation. Inevitably, control over the body, control over environment and events requires the achievement of an equilibrium, not the replacement of one tyranny with another. The principle of ecology must be observed on the cosmic, political and personal level: a harmony of consumption and waste, of growth and diminishment, of birth-making and death-allowing processes.

If the Pill was a metaphor and means of empowerment, it was also a deception that could lead to enslavement. Like many human inventions, it created the illusion that something external to the self could liberate the self. Designed by men, promoted by men, welcomed by men, the artificial and mechanical autonomy it provided inevitably proved to be as ambiguous as the legendary apple of Eden.

Thus, the question of the ancients is translated into new imperatives: not, "Can woman be saved?" but, "Will woman save herself?" And having saved herself, "Can she save herself *from* herself?"

The paradigms of spiritual development proposed by Kierkegaard and Tillich—overlaid on the historical experience of the female sex—suggest that the spirituality of most women is arrested at the threshold of autonomy and ethical maturity. We have already described the obstacles to be overcome and the means for progressing to the second stage, for emerging from heteronomy into autonomy. What remains? What is implied in Tillich's concept of "theonomy," in Kierkegaard's notion of the "religious" dimension? Is the third stage an option or an imperative?

In a contemporary idiom, we might visualize spiritual development as a threefold passage. In the case of women, the first stage—the "heteronomous" existence—is often prolonged, and hence the passage to the second stage can be fraught with exceptional trauma and terrors. Both stages are inevitably marked by a certain inertia and complacency—a "blindness" to self-transcendence, a "spell" that must be exorcised. Liberation, or transcendence, requires a parallel threefold passage:

	Stages of Spiritual Growth		*Passages of Liberation*
1st	I am determined by circumstances, conditioning, authority. Shaped to fit a role, the world makes me. (Heteronomy.)	*1st*	Freedom from external coercion and constraint.
2nd	I take responsibility for myself, I create a world around myself—transmuting circumstances, decisions into personal ego-space, forging connections with other ego-spaces. (Autonomy.)	*2nd*	Freedom from inner compulsions, dependencies, fears.
3rd	I detach myself from my ego-space (it remains intact—the ground of my being, of my sense of identity and confidence). I listen, look to see what larger forces, energies envelop my own. I transcend my ego-space in submitting to, fusing with this larger force. (Theonomy.)	*3rd*	Freedom from "freedom," from autonomy that is not self-transcending.

The passage from the second to third stage of liberation is particularly problematic. It may not, in fact, be an exclusively autonomous process. Although it has roots in the fundamental psychology of developing humanness, it participates also in the realm of "grace," of transcendent power. Bernard Meland observes that, as we come more and more to transcend the "self-assertive" level of freedom, we find ourselves responding and being transformed rather than asserting ourselves. This new level of freedom is an experience that has "the primary characteristic of undeserved gift."[7] It is not a state of being that we can summon or command at will. We are summoned; we are called to it.

In a cosmic sense, Teilhard de Chardin's laws of "inner unification" or "personalization" seem to echo the universal paradigm in the threefold passage we have described. His stages are variations on the same theme:

1. Unification of self within our own selves ("centration," or autonomy).
2. Union of our own being with other beings who are our equals ("decentration," or autonomous relationship).
3. Subordination of our own life to a life which is greater than ours ("super-centration," or worship).[8]

His rationale for the third stage is both naturalistic and theological. Two phenomena suggest that creation is moving toward a transcendent goal: The rise of consciousness and the evidence that mind is gradually subsuming matter; also the increasing "planetization" of humankind, as evidenced by population density, economic and communication links, and the "telepathic" effect of a civilization in which "our thoughts are tending more and more to function like the cells of one and the same brain." A center, a unity, of higher order draws us like a magnet. We have no choice but to surrender and attach ourselves to it.[9]

Thus, the meaning of liberation cannot be summed up merely in the notion of freedom, or self-actualization, or autonomy. Rather it is the acceptance of a commitment to what Lebret has called *dépassement:* "The ability of each human being to overtake or transcend his own limitations and reach a higher level of achievement, perhaps even reaching the level of mysticism."[10]

In religious terms, *dépassement* suggests the capacity for continuous conversion, metanoia, for "passing over" to a new consciousness. The process is never finished, and hence there is a certain dialectical recurrence in the stages of spiritual development. Religion is simply, "the self-transcendence of life under the dimension of Spiritual Presence."[11] Having made one passage to a theonomous existence, complacency can lead to a new heteronomy.

Conscious rejection of, and refusal to participate in, an emerging creative autonomy often spawns a demonic form of heteronomy (in cultural terms, this may take the form of a particularly venomous backlash). Whether it is South African intransigence, or Anita

Bryant's sexual conservatism, or Phyllis Schlafly's political reactionaryism, or Lefebvre's theological nostalgia, the profile is often the same: a hysterical, literal-minded, anathematizing desire to return to archaic heteronomic conditions. The leaders of these movements are themselves examples of personalities immured in a radical autonomy, closed to theonomic/dynamic dimension that they so often appropriate in order to encourage the abdication of the masses from *dépassement*.

So, in a sense we are all unfinished women if we have not reached the third stage. Unfortunately, for many it is an expendable option. Not everyone can accept the transcendent summons contained in all religions—"What must I do to be perfect?" Self-actualization and creative autonomy are worthy and adequate human goals, but we are finite beings. There are potentialities and possibilities that must be sacrificed because of human finitude. Only a theonomous existence can provide a context for this diminishment. As Tillich reminds us:

> Not all the creative possibilities of a person, or all the creative possibilities of the human race, have been or will be actualized. The Spiritual Presence does not change that situation—for although the finite can participate in the infinite, it cannot become infinite—but the Spirit can create an acceptance of man's and mankind's finitude, and in so doing, can give a new meaning to the sacrifice of potentialities.[12]

How can we know when we have arrived at a threshold of theonomy, of self-transcendence beyond autonomy? Normally, these thresholds occur with the onset of crisis: illness, failure, rejection or loss, depression, a challenging task or insurmountable obstacle. These crises summon us to transcend our capabilities, our expectations, even our peace of mind. They interrupt or redirect the momentum of the autonomous self. They are points in life when the soul/self must either expand or contract. Consciousness cannot remain neutral. A decision must be made, consequences accepted. We are never the same afterward.

For many women, children represent the most serious threat to personal autonomy and—at the same time—the most significant bridge to theonomous selfhood. Every woman must decide whether or not, and to what degree, children will be a part of her life.

> It is in process of the "formation" of the other that I am myself formed anew; in that experience of being formed I may often feel torn asunder; old aspects of my self-conception must die in order for my new transformation into selfhood to take place. As a parent I may experience that necessary re-formation of myself in humility, sorrow and joy.
>
> —Penelope Washbourn, *Becoming Woman*

A considerable number of American popular novels and films in recent years have focused on a theme that can only be described as the "demonic invasion of the womb." Children, in various stages of development, and mothers in various stages of vulnerability or violation, have been the principal figures in these parables of possession. One thinks of *Rosemary's Baby, Demon Seed, The Exorcist, Audrey Rose,* and *The Omen.*

What is the significance of this wave of satanic fertility? The fact that the mothers are often divorced, estranged or abandoned certainly suggests the projection of parental impotence and the dissolution of family structures. But another motive, perhaps more subtle, is embedded in the popular theme—woman's rebellion against unwanted invasion by another life. In an age when women have begun to reclaim their autonomy, when the clouds of Victorian worship of motherhood have begun to dissipate, it should not be surprising that many women—*and men*—perceive pregnancy and childbearing, at least subconsciously, as demonic, as a threat to spiritual integrity.

Very few other human experiences—other than prolonged imprisonment and serious illness—threaten personal autonomy as much as the prospect of pregnancy and childbirth. This is a fact that no man has experienced in any existential way, and this may explain the abstract view that men often take of the abortion issue.

To be pregnant, and to allow the pregnancy to come to term, is to permit a process that is alien to oneself to be engaged inside one's body. It is a process that has its own rhythm and structure, its own end, and is essentially impersonal. In the sense in which it mutates one's identity and demands absolute surrender to its teleology, pregnancy and childbirth are "as close to dying as any other human experience."[13]

Is it any wonder that if the pregnancy is unwanted, the fetus should be regarded as an invading organism, a microcosmic beast capable of utmost violation of the human spirit? The stark and instinctual fact is that, at this juncture, women have seldom been capable of rational arguments—they are too overwhelmed with fear; too concerned for their self-preservation.

> Where there is no love she is singularly unsentimental about life. For a great many women a foetus of only a week or two holds no emotional appeal. Death in any case is part of life. Woman, who is so intimately and profoundly concerned with life, takes death in her stride. For her, to rid herself of an unwanted foetus is almost as much in accord with nature as for a cat to refuse its milk to a weakling kitten.[14]

While this may be true on the level of feeling and a characteristic response of a more primitive consciousness, the decision to abort a fetus is a far more rational and complex act in a developed society, particularly when it is a lawful act. Woman is faced with a conflict between her instinctive feelings and the abstract concept of the "sacredness" of life, between her own right to autonomy and self-determination and the right of the fetus to develop unharmed. Centuries of casuistry, dogmatism and myth have created a moral dilemma. In this sense, the possibility of rational choice enhances the very autonomy that women perceive is at stake. Abdication from a decision for or against each pregnancy, or procrastination in making the decision, only increases the risk of self-division that is so harmful to the embryonic child and the guilt that is inevitable in a late abortion.

Female instincts may, in fact, be a better guide to an ethical norm than at first might be supposed. It is well known that female rejection of pregnancy is most acute in the early stages, that it usually lessens as the embryo begins to manifest its presence. To label the trophoblast of the first several days succeeding conception, or the zygote of the second week, or the early embryo as a "human being" is to define life in purely genetic, mechanical and impersonal terms.

The traditional philosophical notion of hylomorphism (the successive endowment of the embryo with vegetative, animal and human "souls") has a certain consanguinity with the existential experience of women. In the early centuries of Christianity, many theologians taught that in its early stages the fetus was animated but not yet "hominized." This view is supported by some contemporary

Christian theologians in a variety of forms. For example, Teilhard de Chardin's law of "complexity-consciousness," which implies that there can be no truly human consciousness without a proper degree of "centro-complexity," an orderly arrangement of an immense number of cells in a closed whole. In this view, the early fetus is not a fully developed human life even in the biological sense, although it contains the potentiality.

Embryologists also point out that many early fetuses—as many as one third of all those conceived—are naturally miscarried: "If we claim that every conception creates a human individual, then we must admit that perhaps one third of all human beings die and their remains are disposed of without benefit of medical care, legal rights, or religious concern."[15]

The question of when life begins is only one aspect of the abortion argument, however. Other questions are also paramount: When *can* fetal life be terminated, and for what reasons? In the case of violent assault? When the female is extremely young? When personal or family integrity is threatened? When mental health may be seriously jeopardized? The moral dilemmas that most of these situations present suggest that perhaps more than any other human phenomenon, abortion is indicative of our "fallen" state. Whichever way we choose, there is some evil. Our complicity in the defensible diminishment of life gives us constant cause for moral humility.

The indeterminacy of arguments on both sides leaves the abortion decision where it belongs—in the conscience of individual women, faced with a reality. A woman can accept or reject even the possibility of contraception as well as abortion, but she can no longer accept a condition in which she makes no decision about these matters. Moreover, her own self-respect and personal autonomy demand that she enter into a process of discernment that exorcises invalid heteronomic imperatives and exposes her own hidden fears and motives to herself. Only then will her decision be truly "free," the act of an ethically mature person.

In the case of a child who is willed and/or accepted, childbirth presents other challenges for women who wish to preserve their autonomy and integrity. We have, in America, evolved a peculiarly barbaric ritual of childbirth:

> The experience of lying half-awake in a barred crib, in a labor room with other women moaning in a drugged condition, where

> "no one comes" except to do a pelvic examination or give an injection, is a classic experience of alienated childbirth. The loneliness, the sense of abandonment, of being imprisoned, powerless, and depersonalized is the chief collective memory of women who have given birth in American hospitals.[16]

The practices routinely followed in this country have a distinctly heteronomic aspect: The woman giving birth is not allowed to be "in control" of the situation. Doris Haire of The International Childbirth Education Association lists some of these practices:

> Withholding information on the disadvantages of obstetrical medication.
> Requiring all normal women to give birth in a hospital.
> Elective induction of labor (without clear medical indication).
> Separating the mother from familial support during labor and birth.
> Confining the normal woman to bed.
> Shaving the birth area.
> Professional dependence on technology and pharmacological methods of pain relief.
> Chemical stimulation of labor.
> Delaying birth until the physician arrives.
> Requiring the mother to assume the lithotomy position for birth.
> Routine use of regional or general anesthesia for delivery.
> Routine episiotomy.
> Separating the mother from her newborn infant.
> Delaying the first breast-feeding.[17]

Women have been conditioned to be passive recipients of suffering as well as pleasure. Their victimization in the childbirth process is a kind of metaphor for their social situation—an existence in which too much within, too much personal autonomy, is surrendered for the sake of a role or code imposed from without. Spiritual maturity demands that women redefine the experience and the metaphor of childbirth by reclaiming their power over its processes, that they transform it into a symbol of their passage from passive victimization to active suffering, to pain and process freely chosen, befriended, for the sake of new life. This is the heart of the theonomous conversion: The acceptance of temporary diminishment—without the sacrifice of autonomy—for the accomplishment of a purpose that transcends the merely personal and subjective.

Parenthood presents a continuous series of these theonomic moments—moments when we must redefine ourselves, redirect our energies, revise our perspective. Children make self-transcendence easier and more difficult. Because they are ours, it is often easier to accept the outrageous demands that life makes in their interest. But also because they are ours, their "strangeness" is a sporadic and inevitable source of pain and anguish. Life with children is a journey into their "otherness," for which we must learn respect and reverence. It is also an unnerving exploration of our own "otherness." In a sense, we do not know ourselves until we have known and been known by children. They reveal us to ourselves in ways that no adult ever could. A mother describes the conflicting emotions that her child evokes in her:

> I am terrified of the power she has to unleash emotions in me, my loving and my raging. I don't think of myself as a violent person, but I know through her that I am. I am horrified at what I can unleash in her—the tantrums, such rage! I live every day with the guilt, the ambiguity, the sense of uncertainty about each of my actions. I want, like every other parent in the world, to be a good parent, and never before has anything conspired to make me feel more inadequate, more anxious and guilty, more insecure. Our poor children. You have the power to destroy all falsity and reduce us to see us as we are, humble us to see ourselves with all our superficial masks torn away! The sight is painful.[18]

Parenthood brings one to the edge of one's identity and tests its authenticity; it even detaches us from it. We get huge doses of pride and humility in alternation. We are tempted "to be as gods" with our children; we struggle to make them our "friends." God himself could not be more catalytic, more apocalyptic in our lives.

This is perhaps why, in the Gospel, children are so closely associated with the "Kingdom," with the transition to a theonomous existence. They are precipitous intrusions in our lives; they are barometers of our own capacity for transcendence. Loving acceptance of them is all that is necessary; righteousness is not a prerequisite.

The image of the child in the Old Testament has a double aspect: that of gift as well as sacrifice, and sometimes that of punishment and expiation. The image of the child in the New Testament likewise has a double aspect: that of exemplar and also sacrament. The twofold significance is illuminated in Matthew 18:

> At that time the disciples came to Jesus and asked, "Who is the greatest in the Kingdom of Heaven?" He called a child, set him in front of them, and said, "I tell you this: unless you turn around and become like children, you will never enter the Kingdom of Heaven. Let a man humble himself till he is like this child, and he will be the greatest in the Kingdom of Heaven. Whoever receives one such child in my name receives me."

It is clear that the New Covenant is antithetical to the Old. Instead of Moses, disciples are urged to imitate the child and to receive the child as a messiah. Jesus seems to emphasize, in these and similar passages, the "otherness" of the child. The core of the Christian ethic is, in fact, an openness to the stranger—the "other," the one who does not think or live as we do, who cannot take responsibility for himself, who cannot always return our kindness. "Anything you do for these, the least of my brethren, you do for me."

The sentimentality which is often glazed over the Gospel words about children obscures the stark existential diminishment implied in those passages. Those who accept children—little ones—into their lives wed themselves in a radical way to mortality. Children do not give us immortality—they teach us to die and to be born again.

May we go mad together, my sisters.
May our labor agony in bringing forth
  this revolution
be the death of all pain.

May we comprehend that we cannot be
  stopped.

May I learn how to survive until my
  part is finished.
May I realize that I
    am a
    monster. I am
    a
  monster.
I am a monster.

And I am proud.

—Robin Morgan, "Monster Poem"

There is, in the present era, a tendency to assume that if there is a passage to higher being, to intensification of life, to a God-encounter, it lies through what have popularly been described as "peak" experiences. Contrary to this view (a stock-in-trade of the "Me-business" and the "self-absorption" industry), authentic spiritual experience suggests that it is more likely to happen when we find ourselves in the "pits." Dostoyevsky once remarked that "One has to be a bit ill to really feel alive." The experience of depression is often a critical threshold in the spiritual life, leading to an autonomous or theonomous transcendence if it is successfully navigated.

Dante's *Divine Comedy,* perhaps the greatest poetic exploration of the spiritual life known to our civilization, begins with the pilgrim soul in the midst of a deep depression. Ciardi's translation reads,

> Midway in our life's journey, I went astray from the
> straight road and woke to find myself alone in a dark
> wood. How shall I say
>
> what wood that was! I never saw so drear, so rank, so
> arduous a wilderness!
> Its very memory gives a shape to fear.
>
> Death could scarce be more bitter than that place!
> But since it came to good, I will recount all that
> I found revealed there by God's grace.[19]

Depression is the most common emotional problem of the 1970s. Women suffer from it more than twice as frequently as men and attempt suicide because of their depression three times more often than men. At the root of this characteristic epidemic among women is an element of self-denial and self-destructiveness. The onset of depression is not always dramatic or even evident. It is often disguised; diverted into other symptoms. One woman confesses that she lived in a state of depression for seventeen years, without really understanding or admitting what her inner feelings were. Esther Harding describes it in psychological terms: "The life energy and interest disappear into the unconscious, and the conscious life is left high and dry, sterile, arid, miserable and *isolated.*"[20]

Because of the diffuse quality of chronic depression (in contrast to a brief period of depression related to a specific event or loss), it is often attributed indiscriminately to a wide range of causes. In the popular mind, any mental aberration in a woman between the ages of 35 to 60—particularly depression—is likely to be attributed to "her changes." The myth of menopause serves as a camouflage for a much more fundamental problem. Two or three definitions provide more practical insight. Freud's view that depression is "anger turned inward" is especially pertinent. In women, the hostility that should be directed outward is often turned in upon the self. The existentialists would prefer to describe depression as the experience of "loss of meaning in one's life." Phyllis Chesler has combined both of these insights in her own analysis of depression as a condition of mourning:

> Women are in a continued state of mourning—for what they never had—or had too briefly, and for what they can't have in the present, be it Prince Charming or direct worldly power. It is not very easy for most women to temper, idle, or philosophize away their mourning with sexual, physical, or intellectual exercises. When female depression swells to clinical proportions, it unfortunately doesn't function as a role-release or respite. For example, according to one recent study, published by Dr. Alfred Friedman in 1970, "depressed" women are even *less* verbally "hostile" and "aggressive" than non-depressed women; their "depression" may serve as a way of keeping a deadly faith with their "feminine" role.[21]

Moreover, she points out further that potentially hostile or aggressive women would gain fewer secondary rewards than depressed women: "their families would fear, hate, and abandon them, rather than pity, sympathize, or protect them." This phenomenon can also be observed in single-sex situations—from female steno pools to religious communities. The profile of the depressed woman is remarkably consistent: feelings of inadequacy, inability to handle conflict and aggressive feelings, a history of martyrdom with no rewards to make up for years of sacrifice, a need to be "needed" in order to feel worthwhile, adherence to conventional expectations, obsessive, compulsive "supermother and superhousewife" behavior. A characteristic trait of depressed middle-aged women is overprotection and overidentification with children. But depression is not a disease only of middle-aged women. It affects college women who are perhaps "trying harder" and not enjoying it, or young career women who are not getting the approval and the rewards they expected.

The pattern that emerges suggests that chronic depression is more likely to occur in those who are too closely identified with a cultural role, in women who live according to the "should system": The should system sets impossible standards for their behavior, and when they inevitably fail to meet those standards the "perfect self" becomes a "despised self."

Depression also tends to be more common among "love-addicted" women who live vicariously through others.

From the perspective of spiritual development, many depressed women are fixated at the threshold of autonomy, of a truly ethical existence; others perhaps, at the threshold of a theonomous or religious transcendence. The latter condition may be characterized more by feelings of ennui and meaninglessness than by personal inadequacy. In a theological sense, depression may be a manifestation of the "sickness unto death" or existential despair described by Kierkegaard. He describes two varieties: 1) the despair of not being able to will to be oneself (the despair of weakness), 2) the despair of willing despairingly to be oneself (the despair of defiance, obstinacy). Thus, within a belief structure, severe depression may, if it is not resolved, constitute a state of *sin*. Kierkegaard clarifies this: "Sin is this: before God, or with the conception of God, to be in despair at not willing to be oneself or in despair at willing to be oneself . . . the factor which dialectically, ethically, religiously, makes 'qualified' despair synonymous with sin is the conception of God."[22]

We must assume, then, that a woman who has accepted a religious faith sincerely has no choice but to resolve depression. It presents, at one or more moments in her life, a "call" to self-transcendence. It requires obedience. When it occurs at the threshold of theonomy, it wrenches us out of our detached autonomy and confronts us with new imperatives:

> One meaning of the experience of depression is that our wholeness, our individuation, the Self, can no longer wait while we follow egotistic ways or even seek for legitimate ego fulfillment, and so the self brings us, drives us, into the wilderness of depression, for God waits in *that* place.[23]

The passage though depression will be marked by a characteristic *irony* and *dread* at the conscious level: Irony makes us aware of the incongruity between our actual and imperfect self and the ideal possibilities of the self. This tension must be invoked if the depressed person is to avoid sinking into an unperceiving, content-less well of emotion. This is the meaning of Kierkegaard's maxim that, "an authentic existence is not possible without irony." He adds that it is necessary to be "rightly in dread" in order to achieve "a healing from the very bottom"; we must maintain an honesty toward our "possibilities" and a recognition of what these possibilities may demand of us. A safe passage through depression requires that we hold our conscious self at a critical distance, and that we befriend our unconscious. It demands a willingness to confront the monster, the beast, the shadow, the emptiness within.

Some women may be diagnosed "mentally ill" for a time. Here again, we are dealing with a phenomenon that frequently appears to be linked to the sex role. Many more women than men exhibit, seek treatment for, and are hospitalized for "psychiatric disease." Schizophrenic symptoms, in particular, are no longer attributed to exclusively biological or pathological causes. It may, in fact, be "a special strategy that a person invents in order to live in an unlivable situation," an abdication from a false outer ego that has been laid on us by others. Thus, clinical explanations of "madness" are being qualified more and more by existential and social considerations. Chesler, for example, relates mental illness directly to sex-role conflict, when she defines it as the acting out of the devalued female role or the total or partial rejection of one's sex-role stereotype.[24] What we see in some people whom we label and treat as psychotics or schizophrenics is in reality the acting out of an experiential drama that can be as much of a breakthrough as breakdown. Gregory Bateson has described the schizophrenic experience—the split between inner and outer world—as a voyage of discovery which, once precipitated in the subject, seems to have an inherent teleology of its own. Those who return from it come back with insights and "possibilities" unknown to those who have never embarked on the journey. He notes, "What needs to be explained is the failure of many who embark upon this voyage to return from it."[25] Clinical and institutional care have largely invalidated and mutilated this kind of experience which is primarily an experience of the soul.

Laing and the anti-psychiatrists insist that we can no longer assume that abnormal behavior and retreat from reality are pathological states. They urge us to recognize that mental illness may be a passage to a happier, more authentic self. In many instances these are processes that should be assisted and guided, not obliterated with electroshocks, tranquilizers, sometimes even with psychoanalysis.

It is not easy to distinguish experience that is "invalidly mad" from that which is "validly mystical." Particularly in the case of women, those who function as their guides must be alert to the social and political aspects of their existence that may contribute to neurotic or psychotic behavior. Neither chemicals nor "adjustment" therapy will cure them of a state of mind that is, at bottom, an act of self-preservation.

The dark night of the soul overtakes us in many ways: through the experience of depression, failure, mental illness, physical illness. They are death-and-rebirth passages to a fuller life. Where does one go for help in navigating these perilous voyages?

> So perverted is the religious element in woman's nature, that with faith and works she is the chief support of the church and clergy; the very powers that make her emancipation impossible.
>
> —Elizabeth Cady Stanton, *The Woman's Bible,* 1895

For many women, religion has led to a perversion of the spirit rather than to its liberation. Sadly, these women are often unaware of the extent of their betrayal of themselves and of the transcendent call embedded in all great religions.

As "woman's sphere" narrowed and constricted more definitely in the nineteenth century, religion became almost the only public role available to energetic women. Moreover, ministers and priests soon recognized that the tidal wave of industrialism had left them a constituency made up predominantly of females. They soon learned to "educate" them, cultivate them and use them to sustain their hegemony. Women's diaries of the period reveal the enormous psychological investment they placed in religious voluntary associations; for the most part maternal and moral reform societies, prayer groups and missionary support organizations. There is no doubt that this involvement held some positive benefits for women, notably the sense of quasi-public identity and, perhaps more importantly, the experience of a community of peers. The negative effects, however, inevitably override these more positive aspects.

It is clear that the socialization of women and their exclusion from significant public roles has made them vulnerable to heteronomic "possession" by clerics and social moralists. Restricted to pious self-expression and auxiliary supportive roles, the "formula female"—destined to be the primary consumer of the spoils of capitalism—is conditioned also to be the primary consumer of organized religion. Excluded from preaching and presiding in the formal ministry of the churches, women become paraffin under the impress of the patriarchal consciousness. Because they are not creative actualizers, women become passive consumptives—sometimes, in the literal as well as religious sense. Women become addicted to, intoxicated by, religion.

The significance of this kind of passive addiction on the personal level will be obvious. In terms of an entire culture, its significance is all the more toxic. As the liberation theologians have so eloquently expressed it, the redemption of society is impossible unless believers are capable of "significative re-expression of the gospel," unless they can be transformed from "gospel consumers" into "gospel creators."[26] Unless women can incarnate religious experience and revelation into the flesh of their present existence and give it new, authentic expressions, the culture itself—in which the *practice* of religion has become so "feminized" and reified—remains sterile. The fossilization and commercialization of religion is only possible in a culture where the devout have not yet discovered the God waiting to be born in themselves. Women, by and large, have internalized an Old Testament transcendentalism that deadens true religious life, a life that, as Berdyaev says, "has degenerated into a police action against the growth of spiritual experience."[27]

The passive-consumptive role of women believers is reflected in a number of distorted relationships. In respect to men, women internalize heteronomic, "received" images of themselves either as seducers or as saviors. In the post-Victorian era, the latter fantasy is probably more prevalent among women with religious affiliations. Women provide moral and spiritual uplift in a masculinized world, they inspire and exemplify the highest human values—men, of course, content with their option on crassness, encourage women in these fantasies by excluding them from their male preserves and prerogatives, even from their language. Because she is essentially alienated from the male world, woman's mythical moral and spiritual influence amounts to little more than the effect a band of cheerleaders might have on the execution of a football game. Cheerleaders do not affect strategy.

The "other-centeredness" of women perpetuates a tendency in them to use religion for therapeutic reasons rather than as a principle of dynamic change and growth. Because they do not see themselves as agents of spiritual energy—as divinized, transcending centers—religious experience becomes something to be applied to oneself, or which one applies to life's hurts; like a poultice. Women see themselves as the chief recipients rather than as dispensers of the healing, celebrating and teaching medicines of organized religion. (At times throughout history, when they have attempted to assume or usurp these functions as agents and dispensers of spiritual alms, they have inevitably been purged as witches, or dismissed as hysterics.) Advice-seeking behavior prevails among women, as we have previously noted. Their need for approval and security generates a doctor-patient relation between clerics and women. (Fueled also by their male mentors' compulsive need to give advice, to play the role of guru—the one with all the answers as well as the "power of office.") This hierarchical, therapeutic relationship epitomizes the patriarchal closure of women, their fixation as the primary votives of sacred dispensation and spiritual direction. If women are to mature in the spiritual life, this unauthentic, non-autonomous pattern of relationship must be broken. Their religious experience is fixated in a kind of Electra complex that must be exorcised. If the patriarchal religions provide little inspiration in this direction, an old Zen maxim does: "If you meet Buddha on the road, kill him!" Woman's failure to take full responsibility for her own spiritual life is a form of idolatry:

> This admonition points up that no meaning that comes from outside of ourselves is real. The Buddhahood of each of us has already been obtained. We need only recognize it. Philosophy, religion, patriotism, all empty idols. The only meaning in our lives is what we each bring to them. Killing the Buddha on the road means destroying the hope that anything outside of ourselves can be our master. No one is any bigger than anyone else. There are no mothers or fathers for grown-ups, only sisters and brothers.[28]

Women struggling to grow up in the spiritual life need fewer priests, ministers and doctors in their lives and more "soul friends." Women, perhaps some men, who can be authentic guides because they are authentic peers—persons of autonomy and transparency who are willing to take the risk of self-exposure who can be fellow and sister pilgrims, in whom there are no traces of the temptation to play Pygmalion, to control and manipulate a soul taking shape.

If the cultic aspect of religion has perpetuated woman in a kind of spiritual infancy, the cosmological aspect has estranged her even from herself. Women, especially, have internalized a concept of God as radically *"Other"* in a double sense. First, God is transcendent, "out there," distant from human experience. Secondly, God is *Male*. Rosemary Ruether calls this "an idolatrous projection upon the nature of the divine of the characteristics of the ruling sexual group in society." She notes the fundamental basis of Christian theology in a "Genesis language":

> It has been axiomatic in Biblical theology that the relation of God to Creation must be defined as that of transcendence and separation of natures. Genesis language that sounds as though the world *flowed* from or was *born* out of God is condemned as "pantheistic." The proper stance of God to Creation is one of a spirit Ego who "makes" the world as an object over against and other than "himself." In other words, the language for genesis is instrumental, rather than the language of gestation. The world is to be seen as something outside of, beneath and other than God. It exists as an inferior and dependent artifact which "He" makes from nothing. It is totally the expression of "His" will and sovereignty.[29]

The affinity of the biblical image of God with male experience is evident. It reflects an instrumental, hierarchical, subject-object relation of "maker" to "thing-made," a "non-participatory concept of creation that makes the world an external object of control and mastery."[30] This image of God as a "transcendent male-mind," who creates an objectified world subject to his sovereignty, provides the model for the way the patriarchal power structure relates to women, children, servants, workers, animal life, property and environment. Reality is split into subservient creatures and transcendent male authority.

The dualism of the biblical tradition was compounded for Christianity by the dualism of the Greco-Roman heritage. The Greek view of reality habitually separated mind and body, thus dividing human rational and carnal capacities (the etymology of "carnal" shows a decided worsening in the writings of the Church Fathers). Carnality acquired an increasingly negative connotation; hence it was assumed that the mind (rational powers) had a "natural" superiority over the body (carnal faculties). This hierarchical duality became the paradigm for all sorts of "natural" inferior-superior relationships (so-called differences between subject and object, self and other, man and woman, master and slave, white and non-white, reason and emotion, ad infinitum). Woman, then, becomes associated with the inferior powers of human nature. Thus, a dualistic secular epistemology and a dualistic biblical cosmology merge in the characteristic misogyny of Western civilization. Eve—woman—because she incarnates inferior energies, becomes a stereotypical source of evil. The Church Fathers propagate a suitable mythology: "Women, do you not know that you are Eve? You are the devil's gateway . . . How easily you destroyed man, the image of God" (Tertullian). There are frequent variations on this theme, like this one from no less a light than Ambrose: "She who does not believe is a woman and should be designated by the name of her sex, whereas she who believes progresses to perfect manhood, to the measure of the adulthood of Christ." To be a Christian one must be desexed—if you are a woman! The flight from sin is equated with the flight from the body and the flight from woman. The path to salvation, toward God, is equated with proximity to, resemblance to, a male archetype. By the year 1140, the *Decretum* of Gratian, the first enduring systematization of church law, could assume with impunity, as most believers did, that "Woman is *not* made in God's image."[31]

Even as late as the 1970s we are witnessing the doctrine of "resemblance" as an argument against women's full participation in the priesthood of the faith. But perhaps even more critical is the mutilation of the spirit which the image of God as Male has wrought in the lives of women. When religious faith demands that a woman masculinize her spirituality and internalize patriarchal models of experience, that faith is unauthentic. For some women, it may even be demonic. Yet, this is precisely what most of the great religions demand of women. How can a woman progress to the higher levels of spiritual experience when approximation to ultimate communion with transcendent Being requires increasing rejection of her own image and nature?

Woman has adapted herself to a relationship with a transcendent Being who is radically Other than herself. The closer she comes to this God, the more she loses her own soul. A woman has no choice but to be an atheist.

> It will be a great thing for the human soul when it finally stops worshipping backwards. We are pushed forward by the social forces, reluctant and stumbling, our faces over our shoulders, clutching at every relic of the past as we are forced along; still adoring whatever is behind us. We insist upon worshipping "the God of our fathers." Why not the God of our children?
>
> —Charlotte Perkins Gilman, *The Home,* 1910

The rejection of a heteronomic image of "God as Father" and the recovery of an autonomous image of God that is experienced as transpersonal, as a "ground of personality," is essential to spiritual maturity. In women it is the most critical threshold of theonomy. It precipitates what Haught has called "the atheistic moment."[32] To resist this moment by clinging to a heteronomous God-image is a way of resisting natural pressures toward self-appropriation. One feels more secure in a world of projected norms; but the threshold cannot be bypassed. Initially, it often manifests itself as a rebellion against a God who has prevented one from "being oneself." It may be a gradual inner realization; it may be a cataclysmic upheaval of one's life. It will often be accompanied by anger and bitterness toward religion in general and the church in particular. In the case of women, it often coincides with the psychological threshold of "consciousness raising," the breakthrough to a desire for authentic personal autonomy. (Here we might underscore the view of the liberation theologians that evangelization is to be identified with the task of consciousness raising.)

What is asked of us is nothing less than an exorcism. The moment of atheism is also a moment of expulsion and destruction of idols:

> The image we fashion of God today, like that earlier one, is in large measure a reflection of underlying attitudes whereby we seek to dispense ourselves from the task of being human beings . . .
>
> If our Christian existence is really authentic, then it must be a continuing journey from atheism to faith . . .
>
> Atheism is a necessary element of our faith.[33]

For many, the "moment of atheism" means the courage to think the "unthinkable," to imagine the "forbidden." God, who has been imprinted in our minds as a transcendent absolute, must somehow be recovered in an epiphany of immanence, of divine self-revelation that shatters our received image. Carl Jung describes a dramatic personal experience of such an illumination. During a period of his life when he was preoccupied with thoughts about the transcendent superhuman majesty of God, he experienced a sudden revelation of the radical "otherness" of Divine Being. He struggled against the thought, but it finally broke through his consciousness and overwhelmed him: It was a vision of an enormous turd falling from a heavenly throne and shattering the sparkling roof of a great cathedral.[34]

The transformation of the God-experience and the God-image may not be quite so dramatic for everyone. But for women it must be just as radical, just as unthinkable. A conversion to matriarchal imagery is often the first and most necessary step. There is a good deal of evidence for this in the fictional, poetic and mystical experience of women. Moments of dramatic illumination, such as that of Nina in O'Neill's *Strange Interlude,* who bemoans the absence of a matriarchal deity, are meant to sound iconoclastic, but, in fact, reveal an intuitive truth about the spiritual psychology of women:

> "The mistake began when God was created in a male image . . . The God of gods—the Boss—has always been a man, that makes life so perverted, and death so unnatural. We should have imagined life as created in the birth-pain of God the Mother. Then we would have understood why we, Her children, have inherited pain . . ."[35]

Likewise, the final epiphany of the heroine in the contemporary musical, *For Colored Girls Who Have Considered Suicide When the Rainbow Is Enuf,* emerging from overwhelming affliction, acknowledging her oneness with nature in a new faith: "I found God in myself and I have loved Her fiercely." The revelations of the mystics are perhaps the most intimate and authentic record of the transformation of the God-image. In the *Revelations* of Juliane of Norwich we find one of the most famous expressions of a popular tradition of the Middle Ages, the theme of "God, our Mother": "As truly as God is our Father, so truly is God our Mother."

> I understand three ways of beholding Motherhood in God. The first is grounded on His creation of our nature. The second is the

> taking of our nature—and there the Motherhood of Grace begins. The Third is Motherhood of Working—in this is a forthspreading without end by the same Grace, in length and breadth, height and deepness.[36]

Juliane's insights have a decidedly androgynous aspect, and in calling Jesus "our true Mother," she envisions the Godhead as a ground of being that encompasses every aspect of the expression of personality.

The theme recurs in the writings of male mystics, also—notably in the teaching of Jacob Boehme (1575–1624) and others, who drew from the Gnostic tradition a concept of a primary female ground of unconditioned Being called Sophia, or Wisdom, which was co-existent with the creating masculine deity. The Gnostic roots of some of these mystical revelations suggest that the "revision" of the patriarchal notion of God is as early as Christianity itself. Instead of a monistic and masculine God, many of the texts of the Gnostic "gospels"—*Secret Book of John, Secret Gospel to the Hebrews, Gospel of Thomas, Gospel of Phillip,* and others—describe God as a dyadic being, who consists of both masculine and feminine elements. Some of the texts equate God as Mother with The Holy Spirit, attributing the maternal element of the Trinity to the Third Person. The fact that these heretical or heterodox scriptures were suppressed in the early Church has been linked to an ecclesiastical suppression of women rather than to dogmatic exegesis. The tradition, however, survived in some orthodox teaching, notably in the works of Clement of Alexandria.[37]

While the Gnostic and later mystical conceptions reflect a spiritual effort to transcend the limiting notion of God as Father, they are nevertheless rooted in an anthropomorphic, androcentric sexual metaphor that constellates being according to certain masculine and feminine qualities. The fundamental dualism in which the religious experience is rooted is not completely transcended. All the same, in the spiritual life, the recovery of a maternal God-image seems crucial to the realization of God's immanence in reality and to the process of rediscovering a "received" faith. The alternative is deepening disbelief. The God of Transcendence, says Ruether,

> . . . is the Lord of an eschatological future that constantly denies its roots in the earth. Apocalypticism and agnosticism are end-products of a male God who establishes his transcendence in end-

> less flights from the body, the woman and the world to the above and beyond. The religion of patriarchy ends in the destruction of the world.[38]

Some women, no doubt, will pass through a provisional stage in which the God-image for them will be unequivocally that of "the Goddess." The radical Otherness which the traditional God-image has represented for them can only be exorcised by its opposite. One woman, surprised and shaken by the discovery of a suppressed hostility in her religious experience, expressed what many women seldom articulate: "I didn't realize it, but I didn't like God. I was often angry with Him, distant. Whatever God was, it was not something personally appealing to me."

The provisional stage in which "the Goddess" is recognized and befriended is an evolution in the structure of belief that often accompanies the recovery of a fundamental self-esteem and personal autonomy. Cole's commentary illuminates this point: "The coincidence of the problem of God and the problem of the self is grounded in this fact: the identity of the self is dependent upon the identity of its God."[39] Thus, women can rediscover and revalue themselves and the ground of their being—God—in the recovery of the goddess myths of pre-Judaeo-Christian epochs. The primitive matriarchal religions and cults differ from Christianity in a number of areas that are critical to the spiritual passage to theonomy. First, matriarchal salvation is open to everyone simply by virtue of a relationship to God; patriarchal salvation is contingent upon an ethical judgment that presupposes a system based on abstract principle. Secondly, the matriarchal experience places value on the material world, which is the model for all creation; patriarchal religion places value in the spiritual, supramaterial world for which reason provides the model. Thirdly, for matriarchal religions, time is cyclical, and the meaning of life is found in earthly existence and in contributing to its renewal; in patriarchal religions, time is linear, moving toward a termination of earthly existence and the entry into a spiritual existence. Meaning is found in contributing to this goal.[40]

Matriarchal religious experience, moreover, provides an antidote to many of the excesses of patriarchal experience: It exorcises archetypal images through a process of renominization; it overcomes transcendent instrumentality in immanence; it derationalizes religious experience through the recovery of mysticism and the "numinous"; it replaces clerical elitism with the authority of the individual; it demystifies transcendent religion by identifying divine power within natural energies.

Perhaps the most important aspect of the recovery of the image of the primordial Goddess is the symbolization that she evokes. The paradoxical phases of her image as Mother/Virgin/Goddess integrate the values of fertility and creativity with death and fidelity to nature; of autonomy with sexuality; of strength with beauty. Since history is the progressive enactment of symbol systems, the resurrection of this ancient and primordial language of being might bring forth alternatives to the phallic, masculinized, mechanized social and political postures of our era. To befriend the Goddess is to restore ecological harmony, to prefer receptiveness and gentle control to fission, fusion and velocity.

Carol Christ has described the emergence of spontaneous "Goddess" recovery groups among contemporary women:

> Women gather in groups to pay homage to "the Goddess" by studying ancient religions, sharing personal visions and inventing new rituals. There are no official ideologies and no Scriptures. There is no magisterium. Reverence for nature, respect for the female body, and a cosmic awareness of the rhythms and energies of life are significant elements in these shared experiences. Many of these groups have revived ancient mythologies from goddess-worshipping cultures; some have consciously aligned themselves with wholesome witchcraft traditions that cultivate intuition, dreams and psychic healing.[41]

But theonomy demands more than the detached autonomy, static immanence and narcissistic separatism that matriarchal religious experience may cultivate if it does not, like patriarchy, transcend itself. The sign of the ultimate religious experience toward which all other forms struggle will surely be the inclusiveness of its symbolism, its power of reconciliation—"*mysterium conjunctionis*"—and its power to release truly spiritual redemptive energies. The first fruit of the truly catholic faith will be the liberation of God.

Pasquier identifies this as the central aspect of religious experience:

> Faith is the readiness to enter into this long process of the destruction—one by one—of our false images of God, in order to allow God to be God . . . At the centre of conversion is the experience that no tabernacle can ever be built, no image of God can ever be

> possessed; but that God is always working at the limit, at the edges, stretching us beyond the today and leading us to learn how to trust and how to love, opening us to a constantly new reality, a new truth.[42]

The patriarchal and matriarchal religious experience must ultimately be transcended. The tradition of the androgyne can be a point of departure, but it is not entirely adequate. As Carol Ochs observes, it too has roots in a dualistic perspective:

> The change in thinking that I suggest is more difficult than a change from "Our father which art in Heaven" to "Our parents which art in Heaven." In other words, the concept of an androgynous God is based on the idea of opposites—but if maleness and femaleness are not opposed to begin with, then the concept of an androgynous God may not prove any more successful in meeting the need for a way of understanding the nature of the Deity.[43]

The passage to theonomy is possible only if we have exorcised the dualisms inherent in anthropomorphic concepts of Deity. Berdyaev notes, "The patriarchal conception of God depends upon the social relationships that exist in the family and it reflects them."[44] Moreover, social relationships based on domination, which exist between human beings, have served as a model for the relationship between man and God. Clearly, the exorcism must take place on the psychic as well as the social level. Elimination of psychological dualisms on the personal level must be complemented by efforts to purge social structures that perpetuate unauthentic relations on the political level. Thus, the religious experience of the New Faith will emerge from two fundamental phenomena: 1) the dynamism and self-transcendence of the person, and 2) the progressive incarnation of this principle in social structures. The problem of evil is the same as the problem of the God-image: "Evil is the past of being . . . God is the future of being."[45] *Dépassement* is the passage to theonomy on both the personal and cultural level. Gregory Baum describes this double confrontation (We have transposed Baum's generic "he" to an equally generic "she"):

> In order to realize herself, woman must face the evil on two fronts, in herself and in the society to which she belongs, and unless she wrestles with evil on both these fronts, she cannot move

far on the way to growth and reconciliation. If she confines her struggle to the evil within herself, she will not be able to discern how much her own spiritual values and her ideal for the community are hidden ways of protecting her social and political privileges. In order to become herself, a woman must be politicized.[46]

The New Faith will abandon the static anthropomorphisms of the past and forge new definitions of the God-who-is-coming-to-be: "God is a continuing inner call within our lives toward authentic solutions."[47] The contemporary transformation in the spirituality of women is a sign and symbol of this greater metamorphosis in the religious experience of humanity. Women are emerging from dependence on a Father-God who supplies all their needs and is the source of law and guilt; they are emerging from a culture-bound, Christ-centered masculine spirituality, which does not answer their own experience; they are evolving a relationship to a creative Spiritual Presence, which comes from within them as well as from beyond. Tillich suggests that the spirituality of the Spiritual Presence transcends the rational and emotional dimensions (the intellectualizing and sentimentalizing of faith that many women are immured in) in an experience that is *ecstatic*. Significantly, he says, the experience of the Spiritual Presence "transcends the alternatives of male and female symbolism," the rational and emotional elements, which usually are attributed respectively to the male and female types.[48] The ecstatic mode of this spirituality should be understood in the exact meaning of the word: as denoting both a concentration of the self and absorption in its powers, as well as a transcendence or transport of the self.

The experience of Jesus Christ is a necessary intermediary in the passage to theonomy. If the self is to find its identity through a relationship with its ideal-ego—its God—the absolute image of God must be relativized. The religion of the Incarnate Son emancipates us from the religion of the Father. We are rescued from the contingency and remoteness of a relation to absolute, transcendent Being, and given "one who is like ourselves," who has shared our existence. We are ransomed from the impersonal Law that we might live compassionately according to the Spirit. Jesus represents the liberated self, the soul claiming its autonomy but living intimately with the Father; renouncing all roles but fulfilling them all in a supremely transparent personality—"a paradigm of selfhood, a dialectical incarnation of God."[49]

Yet Jesus seems to have understood that the Son would also be transcended. His prophetic promise of the Advocate suggests a "developmental" correlation: "There is much that I could say to you, but the burden would be too great for you now. However, when he comes who is the Spirit of truth, he will guide you into all the truth" (John 16:12–13). Preston Cole sees this transcendence and displacement as the fundamental basis of revelation:

> The concept of revelation is also grounded in this understanding of the historicity of the God-concept. Revelation is the dialectic of imagination. The Holy Spirit continually discloses itself through the historical evolution of its image. Through the religious imagination new insight into the implications of Spirit for selfhood is preserved in the evolving image of God.[50]

The passage of the individual to the theonomy of the Spiritual Presence has dramatic parallels with the ancient tradition of the "Third Age." Popularized in its most radical form by the Joachimites of the Middle Ages, the idea has roots that go back as far as Montanism in the second century. In essence, it claimed that a "Third Age" of the Spirit would be necessary to complete the redemption begun by Christ. The most significant formulation of the idea in modern times is found in Nicolas Berdyaev:

> The world is passing through three epochs of divine revelation: the revelation of the law (the Father), the revelation of redemption (the Son) and the revelation of creativity (the Spirit) . . . they are all co-existent. Today we have not fully lived out the law, and redemption from sin has not yet been completed, although the world is entering a new religious epoch.
>
> The third creative revelation in the Spirit will have no holy scripture; it will be no voice from on high; it will be accomplished in man and in humanity—it is an anthropological revelation, an unveiling of the Christology of man.[51]

Berdyaev's vision of the "Third Age" has implications for personal spirituality as well as for the evolution of Christianity. In respect to the individual, he claims that higher creative being is unattainable when God is seen as transcendent to man, and that it is only possible in another stage of religious life, "when God in man is immanent." In cultural terms, the "Third Age" will mean the exodus of humanity from religious guardianship, from a Church that has been more intellectual and physical than spiritual, concretizing itself in institutional structures and dogmatic codes. He insists that the first task of a Christian renaissance, of religious maturity, is "to overcome this heteronomic consciousness." In the new age, humanity will turn "not to the physical but to the spiritual body of the Church." (The continuity of the prophetic view articulated by Berdyaev and those before him is witnessed by the reappearance of similar themes in the contemporary liberation theologians, particularly in Juan Luis Segundo.)

Women are at the center of this spiritual and social transformation. What are the signs that distinguish a woman in the process of authentic liberation? It seems that we can now summarize these in retrospect:

1) As women grow more practiced in decision making and problem solving, their capacity for *ethical choice* will increase. In Kohlberg's paradigm,[52] we will see many more women developing beyond "Stage Four" (moral good is equated with faithful conformity to and performance of social norms, irrespective of the effect on the self) to "Stage Five" (fidelity to autonomous personal commitments and capacity to critique-received values, norms) or "Stage Six" (conscience is able to act in opposition to an authoritative or social consensus concerning correct conduct; moral judgments are "reversible, consistent and universalizable"). Some women will progress to a seventh stage in which the ethical imperative of "doing harm to no one" will be extended by a willingness "to suffer persecution for justice sake"—the ethical standard of heroism, faith and sanctity.

2) Parallel to the development in ethical maturity is a comparable growth in capacity for *religious experience,* for authentic encounter with the "holy." We have described this process in terms of the evolution of the God-image, but there are other relevant interpretations of it—for example, the paradigms of the mystical life such as *The Interior Castle* of Teresa of Avila and the writings of John of the Cross. Teresa's seven mansions of the spirit present many intriguing correlations with Kohlberg's ethical stages. There would seem to be an important imperative here: The necessity of a tandem development in ethical and mystical capacity. Much of the contemporary charismatic phenomena, which may resemble the higher levels of mystical expression, are pseudoexperiences unless grounded in authentic ethical maturity of a comparable level. Historically,

women have been victimized by precipitation into religious feelings that are precociously improper to their level of ethical capacity.

Jim Fowler, whose "life maps" we have previously alluded to, also correlates ethical capacity with other aspects of faith development, notably: patterns of world coherence, role-taking, the interpretation of authority and the process of symbolization. Many of the sociopolitical phenomena associated with "emerging" women suggest that these correlations are significant.[53]

3) The first effect of personal autonomy will be the woman's acceptance of *responsibility for her own inner life.* This will manifest itself in any number of ways: in a withdrawal from "therapeutic" heteronomic relationships with male "guides" and a movement toward peer-oriented support groups; in a rejection of androcentric aspects of Scriptures, dogma and ritual, and the revelation of language and myth that flows out of the personal experience of women. The principle of "detoxification" proposed by the liberation theologians is especially pertinent to the situation of women who, for the most part, have been the chief addicts and consumers of religion in the Western world.

> The Church is suffering from sacramental intoxication. With the nature and purpose of the sacraments largely lost, what was once functional becomes toxic. And as we contemplate how to restore functionality to them, we should not be alarmed to find a clearcut withdrawal from practice of the sacraments. Such withdrawal allows people to put some distance between themselves and the sacraments; to create room for a real process of search . . .
>
> But this "distancing" imputed to secularization is itself a positive thing insofar as it does not eradicate "sacred" terms but rather gives them a human, historical content. For this is the first step we must take in the linguistic revolution that is necessary if the sacraments are to exercise their signifying function.[54]

4) In women who are growing spiritually, the *concept of sin and righteousness* will undergo a radical inversion. "Natural law" arguments will cease to be significant in the formation of personal conscience—unless they can be purged of their culture-bound and teleological biases. Theologies that exalt prudential ethics and regard acts of pride and self-assertion as the capital moral sins will be discarded. The traditional moral hierarchy, which eulogized humility and self-effacement, has been detrimental to women and has

seriously inhibited their ethical development. Too little pride, too little self-esteem and self-assertion are the common sins of women. In an early formulation of this distinction (1962), Valerie Goldstein notes that the so-called "feminine" sins are outgrowths of a basic character structure inculcated by cultural norms. Such deviations as "pride" and "will to power" are somewhat atypical expressions. Women are more likely to be guilty of negative rather than positive assertions, such as triviality, absence of concentration, dependency on others for self-definition, tolerance at the expense of standards of excellence, sentimentality, gossipy invasions of privacy, mistrust of reason.[55]

Ascetic traditions that have, as Baum observes, "enkindled in people the hidden love of death," will be rejected—unnecessary suffering, whether it takes the form of "sacrificial love" or vicarious "atonement," will be morally repugnant to those in the process of liberating themselves. Masochism, in all of its disguised forms, will be uprooted from the psyche. A new understanding of Christian *agape* will exorcise the toxic elements in the received tradition, and at the same time it will require a higher standard of morality than ever before. More than "Do unto others as you would have others do unto you," more than "pray for them that persecute you," the new axiom will require us to "Do harm to no thing and no one (including oneself)"—to act on a higher plane of ecological consciousness, purged of all self-righteousness as well as disguised masochism. Women are especially sensitive to ecological aspects of human identity since their fundamental spiritual experience is rooted in their biological ties with life-giving processes. Their developing moral sense and spirituality will reflect this. With contemporary thinkers like Garaudy, women are coming to realize that sin is not the revolt against authority or pride but the failure to fight against injustice, the desertion of the creative human task.

5) A very crucial passage in the process of liberation will be the *recognition and transmutation of anger*. Women's socialization tends to inhibit their ability to reveal and process their inner rage and bitterness. Its manifestation is often blocked by guilt feelings that mute unacceptable emotions. Depression will often be the most obvious sign of the presence of suppressed anger. Most women over thirty require a modified form of "primal therapy," a support situation in which they can surface the anger, open the doors they have closed off, without fear of being invalidated. If the support situation in-

cludes prayer, a process of healing can be initiated. A major breakthrough is the point at which a woman (most of whom have reason to be angry at men) refuses to blame everything on the Enemy (Man) and recognizes her own complicity in whatever lacerations of the spirit she has suffered. A theonomous resolution of the anger ordinarily results in a compensating effort or project of positively changing the circumstances that provoked the anger. (A bitter, resentful housewife may decide to go back to school or work; a depressed working woman may join a union and work for a change; a frustrated mother may join a women's group devoted to improving child care.) Instead of running away, we go "the other mile" in a constructive effort to change the conditions of our existence. Anger thus becomes the spur to social transformation, and is often the first sign that the Spirit is calling us to "authentic solutions" to the human condition.

> The element of transformation through the Spirit comes by the Spirit's providing a "divine discontent," a force that moves toward the reshaping of communal structures in the direction of greater opportunity, justice, wholeness, and humanity for each of its members.[56]

Anger thus provides an *organic* motivation for social change rather than an artificial abstract rationale. It communicates a Spiritual Presence because it is authentic. Women need to learn to process anger and conflict as part of their developing spirituality, and as life-giving "moments" that can bring about change.

6) Finally, a significant sign of authentic liberation in women will be the convergence of two powerful energies: *politicization* and *contemplation*. Women, healed and whole, will find undreamed of resources in themselves, in the dimension of religious experience as well as in the sociopolitical arena. One of the signs of spiritual authenticity will be the reciprocity, the converging planes of both experiences. Contemporary pathfinders like Hammarskjold have left traces of this new alchemy of the spirit. One of the jottings in his journal reads, "Prayer, crystallized in words, assigns a permanent wave length on which the dialogue has to be continued, even when our mind is occupied with other matters."[57]

A fundamental wisdom of the new age is echoed in the principle of liberation theology that, "In the domain of time, salvation is a 'political' maturity."[58] It means the effort to put all the elements of the universe in the service of the humanization process. It means gradually stripping them of their determinant, compulsive character (in both the physical and moral sense), so that they can be put in the service of liberty. Above all, it means placing oneself in the service of a Spiritual Presence.

Thus, as women find new ways of being-to-the-world, they will of necessity find new ways of praying. The old forms will be discarded. In the past, prayer has been an effort to make contact with a transcendent presence, an inner turning away from oneself and ordinary life and a reaching out toward an invisible, remote Other. With the possible exception of the mystics, this has been the characteristic mode of Christian worship and prayer—a gesture of dependency and obeisance, above all, of separateness. In the contemporary era, many Christians have abandoned the familiar formulas, rituals and postures of prayer for a new form of communion with divine energy. To pray to God is to open oneself to the deepest contemplation of and contact with the self, to be in touch with oneself in every aspect of our being: physical, sexual, emotional, rational, to become aware of our participation in a cosmic, divine-life force, to acknowledge the immanence of God in our becoming. This form of prayer is not a denial of the transcendence of God but a recognition of the extension of the mystery of the Incarnation in ourselves. It is a prayer that does not hold itself remote from where we are, or suspend us in a limbo of inactivity. The contemplation that it requires is also an immersion, a penetration of our decisions and actions at a profound level of moral and mystical awareness. We become our prayer.

New forms of prayer will reflect the new wholeness in women. "Other-centeredness" will diminish, and a new sense of self as microcosm, as ecoself, will encompass the self and all that is not self in a Spiritual Presence. Berdyaev suggests that when the "cult of womanliness" disappears, it will signal the healing of an alienated cosmos. (We have substituted a generic "she" in his original words):

> Woman's rebirth as androgyne will mean her acceptance within herself of the whole of nature, the genuine revelation of humanity as microcosm. In the true birth of the integral woman, both God and nature will be within and not outside her. External objectivity was bound up with sexual fractionization.[59]

The New Faith will be characterized not only by the immanence of the Kingdom in the *political,* but also by a *transcendent* vision of the Cross: a realization that civilization will inevitably fail, and that every successive liberation will require a further *dépassement.* If we are religious persons, this anxiety turns into *hope,* and that hope expressed in words, becomes our *prayer.*

> The reason for the artificiality and rootlessness of the Olympian gods, as of the Jewish and Christian God, is that they are *contrived*—deliberately invented by patriarchs to replace the ancient Great Goddess. Thus the only reality in Christianity is Mary, the Female Principle, the ancient goddess reborn.
>
> —Elizabeth Gould Davis, *The First Sex*

At Montserrat, Lourdes and Guadalupe, the pilgrims still come, streaming daily to those shrines, lighting their votive candles, imploring the intercession of a Virgin-Mother-Goddess. The official Church looks on with a detached reverence for the phenomenon, but with a good many theological reservations. In the space of less than fifteen years, between 1950 and 1963, the Church accomplished the impossible: a near-deification of the Blessed Virgin in the promulgation of the dogma of the Assumption in 1950, followed by a decided demythologizing of her role in the pronouncements of Vatican II.

The two events are symbolic of a tension that has existed in the Church from the beginning between the official magisterium and the faithful, between a rational-theological canon and a spontaneous, non-rational popular belief. The patriarchal elite has always been somewhat mystified by the matriarchal masses; but to their credit, they have responded to this phenomenon, even graced it with the orthodox label of "tradition."

Most of the Marian dogmas proclaimed by the Church have been responses to an overwhelming popular ethos. The declaration of Mary as "Theotokos" at the Council of Ephesus in 431 was a response in part to Arianism; but also to a tidal wave of popular devotion to Mary. The testimony of the masses was marked by torchlit processions in the city throughout the night. When the doctrine of the Immaculate Conception first surfaced in 1140, Bernard of Clairvaux, a learned man known for his devotion to the Blessed Virgin, raised serious objections. In the next century, theologians Thomas Aquinas and Bonaventure likewise questioned the doctrine. But the devotion was allowed to develop and was formally declared as dogma in 1854 and enthusiastically received by the faithful. The 1950 definition of the dogma of the Assumption was another example of the Church finally yielding to—and certainly capitalizing on—centuries of popular devotion. Many respected churchmen objected to the dogma, since scriptural basis was so conspicuously lacking, but tradition and the popular will triumphed once again.

Thus, in contrast to most other popular cults, the cult of Mary has been able to generate credal content in the life of the Church in an organic and integral way. The intensity and continuity of identification with the cult of Mary suggest that the popular ethos has its roots in experience that predates and transcends the Christian phenomenon. The Councils of the Church, in declaring dogmas specific to the Mother of Jesus, have in reality simply rationalized deeply felt, primeval, archetypal experiences of cosmic female energy—experiences of power and deity.

The major goddesses of all pre-existing matriarchal religions seem to share four major characteristics with the Blessed Mother of the Christians: 1) the goddess is the mother of a god, 2) the goddess is the bride of the same god, 3) the goddess is a virgin, but is impregnated by a divine power, 4) the goddess mourns her dead.[60] Thus, the relationship of Demeter and Persephone, Isis and Osiris, Ishtar and Tammuz foreshadow the privileges attributed to Mary: the doctrines of Theotokos, Assumption, Perpetual Virginity. Moreover, the history of art in Western civilization provides overwhelming evidence of Mary imagined in her role as Mother of God, Virgin, Queen of Heaven, Pieta, Mediator of Grace. Isis was one of the more typical prototypes:

> The religion of Isis, the Egyptian goddess, was one prototype of many of the ideas taken over in Christian teaching about Mary. Chastity typified her image and worship. Her priests were tonsured and celibate. Fasting, prayer, vigils and moral renewal preceded the initiation of her devotees. She appeared as a beautiful figure who rose from the sea crowned with the moon, wearing a dark mantle bordered with stars. On the basis of moral renewal of their lives, her devotees were promised prosperity in this life and assurance of life after death. She was above all wisdom, the

> companion of purified souls. When the religion of Isis was defeated by Christianity, much of her power and attraction lived on in the devotion to Mary.[61]

The analogues are numerous; the parallels highly significant. Mary is the supreme imagination of an elemental creative power displaced by the later development of patriarchal myths and structures. She is the Great Goddess resurrected. Briffault notes that by the twelfth century, "the Holy Virgin, called by Albertus Magnus the Great Goddess, had, in Southern Europe at least, well-nigh replaced the male Trinity in the current devotion of the people."[62] As for the North, the Celts, at least, took her to their bosom. When Patrick landed on the Irish coast, tradition has it that "he found the Irish gathered together, worshipping an image of Brigante, the mother of the gods. Patrick of the nimble wit and nimbler tongue soon convinced them that the mother of the gods was really Mary, the mother of God."[63] Everywhere her image was executed in the same symbolic forms once applied to pagan mother-goddess icons. Her image is carried into battle on an imperial palladium as Cybele's once was. Mary is portrayed with a crown of stars and the moon as footstool, as Aphrodite Uranios once was; she carries the ear of corn of the *Spica Virgo;* she is accompanied by the dove of Ishtar; and like many of her sister goddesses, she appears as one who overpowers serpents.[64]

The older tradition that connects Mary with the myth of the Great Mother was, of course, deliberately muted by the Church. The pale, plastered Maid of Nazareth who eventually supplanted the great Theotokos icons of the early centuries was a pale shadow of the vital, powerful, autonomous feminine principle. The diluted Christian image, particularly in Western Europe, emphasized the *passive receptivity* of Mary. Her virginity became, increasingly, more of a reflection of a male quest for a spiritual rebirth freed from carnal femaleness—the antithesis of the "virginity" of the mother-goddesses. Ruether observes:

> Thus official Mariology validates the twin obsessions of male fantasies toward woman; the urge to both reduce the female to the perfect vehicle of male demands, the instrument of male ascent, and at the same time to repudiate the female as the source of all that pulls him down into bodiliness, sin and death. Mariology exalts the virginal, obedient, spiritual feminine and fears all real women in the flesh.[65]

This diminishment of the deific and carnal aspects of Mary's role coincided with her exaltation as a symbol of personified "femininity." Jung, for one, has observed a psychological phenomenon that seems analogous to this development in Mariology: The more remote and unreal the *personal* feminine is, the more intense is the male's yearning for a projection of an "eternal feminine" onto social institutions that assume a maternal character in embracing, protecting, nourishing, approving the individual—from the Alma Mater of the university to the personification of cities, countries, sciences, ideals and perhaps, most of all, the Church.[66]

Thus, in eras and cultures where male power has dominant sway, there is a tendency to romanticize a feminine principle. It should come as no surprise, then, that the zenith of Mariological development and the emergence of the dogma of the Immaculate Conception (thirteenth to seventeenth centuries) coincided with the outbreak of witch hunts that took the lives of upward of one million women. Nor should it come as any surprise that in the years following World War II we had another burst of Mariological, "eternal feminine" ideology. (Gertrude von le Fort, et al.) These were the years when women were being advised to leave the labor force to return to the home and devote themselves to motherhood and the care of husbands. It should come as no surprise that in the midst of all this social mythology, Rome defined the dogma of the Assumption in 1950; in 1954 we had a Marian year. These events were not really signs that women were coming into their own in the church, in the immediate sense. Rather, a sign that the church had turned away from real flesh-and-blood women, and like society, was spiritualizing the limitations of her condition. Women could move *up* or *down,* but not laterally into society. (Woman could be assumed into heaven or damned into hell, but she had better not try to take a man's place on the assembly line or in management!)

Alternative images of Mary are emerging in the contemporary era: images that restore her identity with the Goddess myths of power and cosmic fecundity; images that celebrate her association with the poor and the oppressed, the "anawim"; images that illuminate her eschatological symbolism. As an archetype of the religious community in time, of all those who yet expect the appearance of "God with us" and the fulfillment of our collective destiny, she personifies the whole process of salvation history in humanity.

In a special way, she is symbolic of the passage to liberation which is occurring in women today. Her own personal and historical role has been transformed into one that transcends time and place, even as women are acquiring power over their own history and over the events of their own time. The stark scriptural allusions to her presence sketch the outline of a spiritual passage from heteronomy to autonomy: in her willingness to accept the Word of God from an "unorthodox" intervention in her life, in her initiative in eliciting acts of redemptive power, as at Cana. Her presence before the Cross suggests the theonomic transcendence that completes, over and over again, the life of God in us. Her virginity is thus restored to its ancient symbolism of radical personal autonomy, particularly of female autonomy, liberated from procreative necessity. As one who sums up all roles in herself—virgin, mother, bride, bereaved one—she becomes the eschatological symbol of humanity freed from the tyranny of roles. Her prophetic autonomy goes before the community of faith as a pillar of fire in our exodus from nature and necessity. All the dogmas that the Church has declared as her prerogatives—Perpetual Virginity, Immaculate Conception, Assumption, Mediatrix, Mother of God—are in reality humanity's aspirations for itself, for its release from powers of darkness and liberation into light and life.

She is the One who has first given birth to herself, and thus brings forth God among us.

Her embrace of Elizabeth initiates the sisterhood of those who are divinizing the world.

This is the meaning of women's final liberation—that God is being born in each of us.

Art speaks these truths more eloquently than words in a small fifteenth-century wooden statuette, the "Vierge ouvrante" of Cluny. The statuette depicts the Virgin with Child, holding in her left hand the orb of the earth. The statuette opens, however, with the Virgin herself unfolding like a tryptich—inside, images of God the Father, God the Son, the communion of Saints, the entire cosmos.

"The Goddess is once more, as she ever was, the creatrix of the universe, *the self-revealing energy of the unknowable God.*"[67]

Mary is finally the anti-myth—the one who contradicts the fairy-tale heroines "still dreaming through the dreams of men." She has tamed the Beast, she has broken the spell.

the legend

The frog is an amphibian . . . that is an animal with two types of life, a fishlike life as a tadpole and a (predominantly) land life as a frog. This animal, therefore, is an excellent symbol for the gradual metamorphosis from one world to another, or for a messenger from the sphere of the more fluid soul-world to the solid, material world.
—Julius Heuscher, *Psychiatric Study of Fairy Tales*[1]

My guilts are what
we catalogue.
I'll take a knife
and chop up frog.

Frog has no nerves.
Frog is as old as a cockroach.
Frog is my father's genitals.
Frog is a malformed doorknob.
Frog is a soft bag of green . . .

At the feel of frog
the touch-me-nots explode
like electric slugs.

Slime will have him.
Slime has made him a house.
—Anne Sexton, "The Frog Prince"[2]

In a way this story tells that to be able to love, a person first has to become able to feel; even if the feelings are negative, that is better than not feeling. In the beginning the princess is entirely self-

centered; all her interest is in her ball. She has no feelings when she plans to go back on her promise to the frog, gives no thought as to what this may mean for it. The closer the frog comes to her physically and personally, the stronger her feelings become, but with this she becomes more a person. For a long stretch of development she obeys her father, but feels ever more strongly; then at the end she asserts her independence in going against his orders. As she thus becomes herself, so does the frog; it turns into a prince.

—Bruno Bettelheim, *The Uses of Enchantment*[3]

Frogs appear in fairy tales with characteristic impertinence. As with snakes, their appearance usually provokes negative responses of fear, disgust and confusion, especially when they manifest humanlike capacities for communication and relatedness. The hero or heroine recoils from this cold-blooded, amphibian creature that emerges from bogs and ponds, all wet and slimy, and intruding itself in the normal run of things. In a fairy tale, the appearance of a frog is like the advent of a comet in the cosmos—it disturbs and alters the course of every planet or star in its path.

The most popular of the frog fairy tales is, of course, the story of *The Frog Prince*. In Grimm's version (sometimes called *The Frog King*) a beautiful young princess plays with a golden ball which accidentally rolls into a pond. A frog tries to befriend her and retrieves her ball after he extracts a promise from her to allow him to play, eat and sleep with her. The princess soon forgets her pledge, and leaving the frog behind, returns to the castle. He follows her and demands that she honor her pledge. She is repelled, but her father, the king, insists that she keep her promise. The princess is progressively overcome with anger and disgust as the frog intrudes more and more in her life. When he demands to sleep with her, she rebels and in a fit of outrage and revulsion, she smashes the frog against the wall of her bedroom. In that moment, the spell is broken and the frog is transformed into a magnificent prince—a worthy spouse for the princess.

From a conventional point of view, the tale is a parable of puberty and the first experience of sexual encounter. The golden ball, like most "golden" things in fairy tales, represents the higher, spiritual aspect of the personality. In the context of this tale it is also an emblem of youth and innocence, of virginal freedom. The frog is symbolic of the impatient manifestation of physical instincts and the temporary submersion of the spiritual aspect in adolescence. At first the heroine is incapable of integrating the two dimensions of experience, the spiritual and physical. She tries to recapture the golden world while rejecting the ugly frog. The frog persists, grows progressively more intimate: first conversing with her, then playing with her, sitting with her, eating with her, and finally demanding to sleep with her.

The frog's phallic, assertive qualities identify it as an obvious projection of male sexuality. In an earlier version of the tale, the significance is even more explicit: the princess must kiss the frog while it lies in bed with her, then they must sleep together for three weeks before the frog is transformed into a prince.

Feminists might well object that the conventional interpretation of the tale is a cautionary message to females to bear with the atavistic aspects of the male personality, to accommodate themselves to the abrasive, exploitative demands of a male partner. The patriarchal, androcentric bias of the tale is underscored by the fact that the heroine's accommodation is prescribed by her father, the King. The all-too-familiar pattern of the battered woman is evident: initial anxiety, anger and hatred are gradually pacified by the realization that she has nowhere to go, no one to turn to. Her isolation and dependency make her a prisoner of male will.

Another evidence of the veiled androcentric-misogynist bias of the fairy tale is the curious epilogue that is often added to the story, a brief passage that celebrates the loyal devotion of Iron Henry—the frog prince's faithful servant—to his master, in spite of his changed form. Presumably, Henry's faithful and heroic love is introduced as a deliberate contrast to the unfaithful princess who defaults in her promise of friendship to the frog. The male comrade provides the exemplary image of love, rather than the female consort.

But the denouement of the tale suggests a more universal meaning. Both the princess and the frog are destined to be changed. At first the princess obeys her father, but her anger and outrage intensify, finally liberating her personality from the father-image (superego) in an act of self-assertion. "As she thus becomes herself, so does the frog."

The frog, too, must be liberated from his obvious need to achieve a symbiotic dependency on the princess. He must experience being thrown out of her bed and hurled against the wall. He must experience being reduced to nothing—ignored and finally annihilated. Only then is the frog "freed of bondage to an immature existence."[4]

Thus the tale of *The Frog Prince* celebrates not only the integration of the spiritual and the physical in the sexual encounter, but also the achievement of personal autonomy and the maturity of relatedness. The amphibious nature of the frog highlights its significance as an intermediary between two worlds; even as sexuality mediates the physical and spiritual dimensions of the personality and constitutes a crucial passage to psychological and spiritual maturity.

The fact that many variants of *The Frog Prince* reverse the sexual roles and focus on a "Frog Princess" suggests an even more universal symbolism. In the Russian tale *I Know Not What of I Know Not Where,* the Tsar's archer can only retrieve his golden-haired wife by riding on the back of a huge frog that leaps across the river of fire into the "I Know Not Where Land," and by finding there, "I Know Not What," who helps him defeat his enemies. Likewise in *The Frog Princess* the hero finds his wife's frog skin and burns it. For this impulsive act he is punished: the frog-princess leaves him and warns him that she can only be his again if he is willing to search for her "beyond the thrice ninth land, in the thrice tenth kingdom." Ivan, the hero, seeks her in a land of darkness, mystery and oracle. After several years and much toil, he finds her and frees her from her enchantment.

The symbolism of fire in both of these tales represents an act of self-destruction, an assumption of absolute control over a vital dimension of one's being that is subsequently punished by its loss and painstaking recovery. The juxtaposition of *The Frog Prince* and *The Frog Princess* tales suggests that what has been rejected or lost is some part of the soul or psyche that is integral to the whole person. Jungian psychology provides an apt, if somewhat particular, interpretation: in *The Frog Prince* the heroine has rejected her own animus qualities, and in *The Frog Princess* the hero has obliterated his anima. In a more universal context, the variants of the tale suggest that the frog-persona represents whatever has been suppressed by reason of social role. Only in the relationship of human love is the bond secure enough, elastic enough to withstand the eruption of those aspects of the person that have been muted by the tyranny of culturally imposed roles. Men and women need each other.

The Frog Prince, especially, has a unique contemporary resonance as a parable or metaphor of the crisis of identity in the relations of men and women. Women in the process of shedding the "feminine mystique" and discovering an authentic self, are progressively repulsed by the conventional masculine role. The more macho a man is, the more of a frog he is. The more a woman is liberated from stereotypical roles, the more unacceptable he becomes. But a man may insist upon sharing a woman's private, intimate life (even as she has begun to demand a share in his public, social life). He may pursue her, force his participation on her; she cannot escape some ultimate engagement with this frog-persona.

It comes first in her submission to the patriarchal authority of the masculine view of reality. In time, her own rage, anger and depression may free her from this father-ordered cosmos. She undergoes a metamorphosis of consciousness. She exorcises the patriarchal hegemony in her soul, discovers a new identity. Suddenly, her partner begins to resemble a frog. What has she done, what alchemy of the spirit has transformed him into an ugly, surly toad? But he does not see himself as a frog—he does not comprehend at all when she tries to explain how she sees him. She has no choice but to take the risk of rejecting him—of leaving him or throwing him out, reducing him to nothing. In that moment of truth, he has a choice. He can commit himself to the arduous pilgrimage of transformation, toward gaining a new vision of himself; or he can sink into self-pity and remain fixed in his blindness. He may go on forever mimicking the compulsive, false premises of that original relationship. He may never know that he is a frog. After all, the woman has cast off an alien image; he is being asked to murder his own self-image.

Metamorphosis cannot take place without the rupture and shedding of old shells and old skins—of conventional structures and traditional roles. But we are afflicted with a mortal inertia, men and women alike. The transformation may never come. Many will rot in their chrysalis and never know sunlight, airy winds and freedom.

EPILOGUE

Exit the Frog Prince

Dearest Prince,

I have not quite decided whether I should leave you. I know you are confused and anxious. You keep looking at me with that "whatever-happened-to-the-princess-I-married" look. Your confusion is understandable. In the past few months, years, I have literally self-destructed. Disintegrated my false self, in order to reassemble my true self. Your self, unfortunately, is tailor-made for that old, false self. You are accustomed to playing "hero"; suddenly you're a "heavy."

Like many other men, you have difficulty seeing yourself as an oppressor because you have difficulty seeing yourself as a member of a class. Men regard themselves as individuals and look to their own motives to justify or reprove their behavior. They suppress their symbolic role in an apolitical illusion of personal innocence: "I have never discriminated against women or bullied them, so why should I be accused?" They are blind to their participation in sustaining oppressive arrangements in human relations. They have accepted the way things are, and in that acceptance is an act of complicity—regardless of their own personal motives. Their individualistic view inevitably seduces them into interpreting efforts to redress the situation of women—"affirmative action" plans, etc.—as threats to their own individual rights. The hue and cry about "reverse discrimination" is a pathetic wail of self-centeredness as the last lifeboats on the *Titanic* are loaded.

In working through my own liberation I have experienced much anger and a great deal of fear. But I am beginning to emerge on the other side of that, now. I can begin to look beyond myself to be concerned in a new way about others. My anger has changed to anguish —anguish especially about you. In so many ways, your situation is worse than mine. Your self-deception is deeper and more profound.

I know you instinctively regard the "woman problem" as a question of giving them time and space enough to "catch up" with men. You don't see yourself as having a problem, too. White, middle-class American males always think that everything is someone else's problem—the blacks have a problem, women have a problem, chicanos have a problem. You don't recognize your own socialized masculinity as a problem, as the root of all the other problems.

In a sense everyone's liberation depends on the liberation of white males, precisely because they have the power to prevent women and minorities from seeking a broader range of alternatives if they do not play the game by the rules of the masculine value system. Unless you can admit that you *are* the problem and begin the task of liberating yourself and dismantling the male-ordered system, many so-called "liberated" women will be seduced into a patriarchal, elitist, one-dimensional, masculine role. We will simply have a new set of "half-persons" who happen to be female.

In many ways, you are more fragile than I. I know if I leave you, it will crush you beyond anything I will suffer. By being a good wife, mother, mistress, servant, handmaid, Girl Friday—and little else—I've made you all the more dependent on me for your sense of well-being. The impression of autonomy that you project to others is a well-practiced reflex. But you are not a truly free person. The heteronomy I struggle with binds me primarily to persons and to the demands they make on me. The heteronomy you have to exorcise is more abstract, insidious and pervasive. Independence will not necessarily free you to the extent that it will free me. I had to recognize that I had no being of my own. You have to recognize the extent to which your being is dependent on affirmation by women and by your "inferiors." Your dominance, your assumption of the natural superiority of the male sex, is really an attempt to guarantee the continued presence of those on whom you depend for your identity as a male.

As women, we are constantly made aware of our immanence, of our contingency, of the social and biological parameters that circumscribe our being—we need few reminders of what it means to be female. Men, on the other hand, enjoy a more individuated transcending role. Thus, their awareness of their masculinity—in a patriarchal society—requires the recognition and confirmation of their supremacy. One can't be a Chief unless there are Indians who provide evidence of it, willingly or unwillingly.

The masculine role is at the same time more restrictive, more abstract and more artificial than the feminine role. Liberating yourself from it will perhaps be more difficult than my exodus from the feminine mystique. Girls grow up with a greater exposure to a same-sex parental model than boys. In the relative absence of his father and care-taking male models for direct imitation, a boy absorbs a culturally rather than concretely defined masculine role: from his mother and teachers, from his peers, from television and other sources of conventional stereotypes. Thus, the role is more abstract and more demanding, more total and more distorted. Deviations from it are more critical; dilemmas abound. Being a man demands independent, aggressive, physically active, ambitious behavior. Educational and societal values tend to be more feminine, emphasizing politeness, obedience, passivity, cleanliness, etc. These double-binds increase as a boy changes into a man, intensifying inner stress and conflict. Growing up male exacts a terrible price, ultimately requiring capitulation to the absolute heteronomy of the masculine ideal.

As a conditioned male you must undergo a mutilation of spirit that amputates some of your deepest human capacities. Feelings are perhaps the most serious threat to the masculine ideal. You are expected to play the role of the independent strong achiever, always in control, always deliberate, calculated. You are expected to be task-oriented, undistracted by personal matters. You are expected to repress any responses that might impede your efficiency in achieving your goals. And so you listen neither to your feelings, nor to your body. You do not sense the approach of illness or register the whispers of your own mind. You often do not hear what others are trying to say; you translate non-verbal messages poorly. Your belief in your own self-sufficiency makes you resistant to the idea of seeking help from someone else. Physically and emotionally, you ignore the pain that signals your innermost desire for health and growth. Not surprising that some psychologists compare the behavior of many men to that of autistic children: the characteristic fear of being touched, of expressing feelings, of relating intimately, with a compensating fixation on inanimate objects.

Sometimes you show very little respect for words; you are impatient with the process of communication and reflection. Your muteness and your silence are often testimony to your worship of will and action. You say you thrive on competition. I'm not so sure. All I know is, it drives you to do things you wouldn't do if you were in your right mind. Sometimes you even compete with your own kids.

In subtle ways you consistently invalidate the experience, the tasks of women. You play the "professional" and demand freedom from simple human tasks—at the cost of your humanity. You hide from life through "specialization." You want your work to be an escalator to success with as few deviations as possible. Oh, I envy your confidence in yourself. But I know it's only skin-deep. You're sure of yourself in the few roles—jobs you've mastered. Left without them, you collapse like a jellyfish in a heap of inadequacy. You haven't learned the art of living. You wear a public face easily, but you're very insecure in intimate situations. You know what mask, what language to use when, but you're out of sync with your inner self.

I would like to free you of your compulsive workaholism, your "breadwinner" fixation. But I can't share that load unless you relieve me of some of the burden of homemaking and child rearing. Can you learn to work less, earn less, spend more time with the kids—and be happy? If you can't, then I can't be happy either. Can you stop measuring yourself by the size of your paycheck?

I want to be an equal partner with you in supporting our home and in building a world. I think I should work, but I don't want to betray myself in "liberating" myself into the marketplace. I know I have to learn how to cope with competition. But I don't want to be infected with it, as you are. If my professional advancement is going to depend on conforming to the male model of achievement (compulsive-accretive production, narrow specialization, manipulation of data, the ability to walk over others on the way up, "chutzpah" and hustling, a cool and stoic demeanor), then I would be a fool to remake myself in your image.

Your institutions are like your automobiles—extensions of your ego. So pervaded by the masculine consciousness that they have become lethal instruments, harmful to all forms of human life. Your hospitals, schools, universities, governments and churches are all corporations, factories. All in bondage to the idea of male supremacy, that might makes right and wealth dictates policy, where workers are excluded from ownership and decision making, and profit becomes synonymous with survival. Most of your institutions are still modeled on the plantation—a few privileged white-male professionals supported by a huge substructure of underpaid, underprivileged, largely female labor force.

When I work in these institutions, I have to endure high visibility as a woman and low visibility as a professional and as a person. My comments are frequently ignored at committee or board meetings. But if you make the same proposal a few minutes later, it's accepted enthusiastically. You are conditioned to notice my face, figure, clothes, manner, but have very little talent for observing and judging capacity. In fact, you are exceptionally stupid when it comes to making judgments about women. Probably because you prefer to surround yourself with "safe" types who will not attempt to challenge or change anything. The fact that they often turn out to be incompetent or lacking in conviction seems to have escaped you.

I'm tired of cloaking my competence with a veneer of coyness—so as not to castrate my male peers. I'm tired of having to let you win—whether it's in checkers or politics. Do I have to spend my entire life coddling male egos? (High school and college were a prolonged ordeal of this kind of dishonesty.) When are you going to recognize your paranoia of competent, assertive women for what it is? An infantile reflex against Mom. *Look* at me: I'm not your mother, your older sister, your baby sister, your first-grade teacher, your servant, or your pet—I'm your *peer*. I'm a *person*.

I'm tired of lobbying for shared responsibility, equal pay, promotions and job opportunities. Women have always wanted these things, unless they've been brainwashed beyond repair. We won't get these things, however, until men realize that *they* have to give up something—power, advantage—in order for us to be equal. Until you promote women's liberation, there won't be any. It isn't going to happen by natural evolution—your present position is too comfortable. You play the "anointed" role, as if authority always had to be given to the oldest son. It might be easier to take if you simply acknowledged the lust for power and the insecurity that underlies your need to be in charge. But you keep referring your status to some fundamental principle of cosmic order, or worse yet, as "God's plan for the human species." The possibilities of human destiny, human structures and human relationships are infinitely more varied than this. Stand back and let the future unfold.

But let us not be naïve. The mere presence of women in new

jobs, in management positions—in greater numbers—is not necessarily going to make a difference. Misogyny and patriarchy run deep, in women as well as men. Much more fundamental changes in social structures are needed if human persons are to develop to their full spiritual maturity.

The look on your face tells me I am guilty, too. Yes, I hate myself for the subtle ways in which I seduce you into being a traditional male—how do we unlearn these old scripts? How can I begin to show you that your personhood means more to me than your masculinity? Will the world around us still convince you otherwise?

I am torn between my resentment of your protective paternalism and the real need I have of the security of your love, your help and your confidence in me. But please, no more Pygmalion postures. I'm trying to reclaim my responsibility for myself, for my own growth and maturity. If I fail, I fail. On the other hand, I don't like being ignored either. You find it easy to promote, help and encourage—to nurture—other men. But you leave women to their own devices. Your distance forces me to work twice as hard to prove myself.

In countless ways we need each other as models for change. But I don't want to be what you are, and you wouldn't want to be what I have been. Can we become something new together?

I am perturbed by your isolation from other men. Oh, you maintain a certain easy acceptance of each other. You can always depend on your cronies for assistance, commiseration. But you have no really intimate male friends, one or two "soul friends," to whom you could open your heart. Am I the only one you can achieve that kind of intimacy with? That's too much for one person to have to provide.

You seem unwilling to admit the presence of "love" in your relationships with other men. Although I suppose if you did, I might instinctively reflect jealousy or suspicion—I've been conditioned too.

I'd like to have some friendships with other men that don't necessarily involve sex. I know I'm capable of this kind of relationship, but I can't seem to find many men who are. Most of them assume that sex is the terminal point of all relationships. And then there's the problem of your possessiveness and jealousy.

I worry about your influence on our children, on the young people we care for. You treat the boys so differently from the girls. Your hyperanxiety about your son is already affecting him. If you were around more, perhaps your daughter would be better off too.

All of these anxieties and frustrations have brought me to a point of decision about you. My own *anger* and *depression* finally forced me to transform my life. What will it take to transform yours? Is *rejection* the only way to open your eyes? Do I have to leave you, abandon you to your self-serving universe? If we go our separate ways, there will be pain and loss. The tapestry of relationships that we have woven with our lives will be rent. If we remain together, we may succumb to the bribes of our old way of life and be diminished that much more. Either way there is risk.

Change will no doubt be more precarious for you than for me. It will be a more lonely, more alienated path. In shedding the husk of your reflected masculine glory, you will discover what many women already know—what it means to be a no-thing. Women in the process of a consciousness breakthrough usually experience rage and frustration. Our behavior is often overtly anti-male. Men undergoing the same process will experience more of a feeling of loss. Anger and resolve motivate a woman to sustain her changed consciousness and evolve new relationship patterns. As she withdraws from male hegemony she will often discover the support and encouragement of other women who will reach out to her in her struggle. You, on the other hand, are likely to suffer the loss, not only of the women to whom you can no longer relate in the old way, but also the loss of your male buddies—because you have betrayed the masculine code. You will be alone, you will be tempted to revert to the old patriarchal and macho scenarios. You have everything to lose by continuing the struggle; I have everything to lose by giving it up.

I want you to know that I understand what is at stake for you. I want you to know that I can support you in that death and rebirth process—it is the price of reclaiming your humanity and your own soul. I can be your companion. My conversion to feminism is an unfinished, incomplete experience unless it leads to your liberation. We can walk beside each other and support each other. We need not be spouses—in fact, it might be better if we weren't. Believe me when I say that I want you to be different (in spite of the fact that I sometimes behave instinctively to the contrary). If I give up my princess ways, will you give up your princedom?

I know I will have to steel myself to accept the consequences If you begin to take on more responsibility for home and children, I will have to sacrifice some of my matriarchal prerogatives there. If you begin to shed the "team" mystique at work, take a stand on sensitive issues, work fewer hours, I will have to bear with the consequences in loss of promotions, lower pay, job changes, whatever may come. I'll have to bear with insecurity and loss of status without putting guilt on you. You'll have to stop putting guilt on me for abandoning the "imperial motherhood" role in the home and the Girl Friday role in the office.

Perhaps the most difficult change of all will be admitting that neither of us can be all things to the other. If we are married, we will have to allow others to be a part of our lives, individually and together. We will need more than other supportive couples, mirror images of our own dyad. I will need women and men as friends; you will need men and women as friends.

We have to be committed to this transformation. These changes will come slowly and painfully. We will have to bear with different rhythms of growth in each other. We will have to persevere in them in spite of the pressures of society. We will have to explode and upset our life together, occasionally, in order to find new ways to keep ourselves growing. This commitment to each other's liberation and growth should be our best reason for being together. If that is not a part of our continuing compact, then even if I love you, I *must* leave you.

You came into my life once and awakened me from sleep, rescued me from servitude, led me through the forest safely. I can do nothing less for you. Can we walk out of the fairy tale into the future together?

With love and hope,
Sleeping Beauty,
Snow White,
Cinderella,
Goldilocks and
Beauty

NOTES

THE LEGEND

1. Simone de Beauvoir, *The Second Sex* (New York: Bantam Books Inc., reprint, 1970), pp. 271–72.
2. Bruno Bettelheim, *The Uses of Enchantment* (New York: Alfred A. Knopf, 1976), p. 234.
3. Marilyn French, *The Women's Room* (New York: Jove Publications, Harcourt Brace Jovanovich, 1977), p. 642.

CHAPTER ONE

4. Margaret Mitchell, *Gone with the Wind* (New York: Macmillan Co., 1945), p. 79.
5. Dory Previn, "Left Hand Lost," from album *Mary C. Brown and the Hollywood Sign,* United Artists, 1972.
6. Daniel Sugarman, Rolaine Hochstein, *The Seventeen Guide to You and Other People* (New York: Macmillan Co., 1972). See also, *The Seventeen Guide to Knowing Yourself* (New York: Macmillan Co., 1967).
7. Enid Haupt, *The Seventeen Guide to Your Widening World* (New York: Macmillan Co., 1965), pp. 24–25, 67–69.
8. Marabel Morgan, *The Total Woman* (New York: Pocket Books, 1976), p. 112.
9. Gabrielle Burton, *I'm Running Away from Home, But I'm Not Allowed to Cross the Street* (New York: Avon Books, 1975), p. 23.
10. F. Scott Fitzgerald, *Tender Is the Night* (New York: Charles Scribner's Sons, 1933), p. 55.
11. Phyllis Chesler, *Women and Madness* (Garden City: Doubleday & Co., Inc., 1972), pp. 33–35.
12. De Beauvoir, op. cit., pp. 45–46.
13. Study by Elizabeth Oleshansky on "Self and Other Orientation: A

Research into Women's Personality Characteristics," unpublished, Michigan State University, 1974. See also Jean Baker Miller, *Toward a New Psychology of Women* (Boston: Beacon Press, 1976), Ch. 6 and 8.

14. Miriam Bar-Yam, "Cultural Differences in Sex Role and Moral Development," Boston University, 1974, unpublished.

15. Gail Sheehy, *Passages, Predictable Crises of Adult Life* (New York: E. P. Dutton, 1974), pp. 293–94.

16. Soren Kierkegaard, *Either/Or* (Garden City: Doubleday Anchor Book, 1944; reissue 1959), Vol. II, pp. 259–61.

17. Paul Tillich, *The Protestant Era* (University of Chicago, Phoenix Books, 1973), p. 46; *The Eternal Now* (New York: Charles Scribner's Sons, 1963), p. 90ff.; *The Dynamics of Faith* (New York: Harper & Row, Pub., World Perspectives series, Vol. 10), Ch. III, "Symbols of Faith."

18. Paul Tillich, *Systematic Theology,* Vol. I (University of Chicago Press, 1963; reissue 1973), p. 84.

19. Paul Tillich, *The Religious Situation* (New York: H. Holt & Company, 1932), p. 39.

20. Jim Fowler and Sam Keen, *Life Maps: Conversations on the Journey of Faith,* ed. Jerome Berryman (Waco, Tex.: Word Books, Publishers, 1978).

21. Kate Chopin, *The Awakening,* in *The Storm and Other Stories* (Old Westbury, N.Y.: Feminist Press, 1974).

22. Sigrid Undset, *Kristin Lavransdatter* (New York: Alfred A. Knopf, 1923; reissue 1937), pp. 992–93.

THE LEGEND

1. Dorothy Jongeward and Dru Scott, *Women as Winners* (Reading, Mass.: Addison-Wesley Pub. Co., 1976), p. 56.

2. Andrea Dworkin, *Woman Hating* (New York: E. P. Dutton & Co., Inc., 1974), p. 41.

3. Bettelheim, *Uses of Enchantment,* p. 203.

4. Joseph Rheingold, *The Fear of Being a Woman: A Theory of Maternal Destructiveness* (New York: Grune & Stratton, Inc., 1964), pp. 136–37.

5. Anne Sexton, "The Double Image," in *To Bedlam and Part Way Back* (New York: Houghton Mifflin Co., 1960), p. 61.

6. Bettelheim, op. cit., p. 211.

7. New Catholic Encyclopedia, on "Original Sin."

8. Marie-Louise von Franz, *Problems of the Feminine in Fairytales* (Middlesex, Eng.: Spring Publications, 1972), pp. 54–55.

CHAPTER TWO

9. Hans Sebald, *Momism, the Silent Disease of America* (Chicago: Nelson-Hall Co., 1976), pp. 52–53.

10. Rheingold, op. cit., p. 2.

11. Nancy Friday, *My Mother/My Self* (New York: Delacorte Press, 1977), pp. 56, 80. Both quotes are from a "Dr. Sanger."

12. Ibid., p. 58.

13. Ibid., pp. 26, 400.

14. Ibid., p. 244.

15. Chesler, *Women and Madness*, p. 18.

16. Marc Feigen Fasteau, *The Male Machine* (New York: McGraw-Hill Book Co., 1974), p. 17.

17. Margaret Mead, *Male and Female* (New York: Mentor ed., 1949), p. 214.

18. Ann Schoonmaker, *Me, Myself and I* (New York: Harper & Row, 1977), p. 38.

19. Shirley Sugarman, *Sin and Madness, Studies in Narcissism* (Philadelphia: Westminster Press, 1976), p. 34, ff.

20. De Beauvoir, *Second Sex*, p. 513.

21. Helmut Schoeck, *Envy, A Theory of Social Behavior* (New York: Harcourt, Brace & World, 1970), p. 166. Trans. Michael Glenny, Betty Ross, pp. 27, 57–58.

22. Ibid., p. 50.

23. Ibid., pp. 22, 225.

24. Ibid., pp. 59, 183.

25. Adrian van Kaam, *Envy and Originality* (Garden City: Doubleday & Co., Inc., 1972), pp. 65–66.

26. Soren Kierkegaard, *The Concept of Dread*, trans. Walter Lowrie (Princeton University Press, 1957), p. 55.

27. Soren Kierkegaard, *Sickness unto Death*, trans. Walter Lowrie (Princeton University Press, 1941), p. 83.

28. Liv Ullmann, *Changing* (New York: Bantam Books, Inc., 1977), pp. 172, 196, 251.

29. Lillian Hellman, *Pentimento*, "A Book of Portraits" (New York: New American Library, Signet Book, 1974), pp. 93–94.

30. Charlotte Wolff, *Love Between Women* (St. Martin's Press, 1971), p. 69. See also, Ruth Tiffany Barnhouse, *Homosexuality: A Symbolic Confusion* (New York: Seabury Press, 1976), p. 84. Sacred Congregation for the Doctrine of the Faith, "Declaration on Certain Questions Concerning Sexual Ethics" (Washington, D.C., U. S. Catholic Conference, December 29, 1975). De Beauvoir op. cit., p. 392.

31. Barnhouse, op. cit., p. 158.

THE LEGEND

1. Bettelheim, *Uses of Enchantment,* p. 273.

2. Judith Long Laws, "Woman as Object," *The Second X: Sex Role and Social Role* (Amsterdam: Elsevier Pub. Co., forthcoming).

3. Philip Wylie, *Generation of Vipers* (New York: Rinehart, 1942), pp. 49, 55.

4. Bettelheim, op. cit., p. 239.

5. Ibid., p. 270.

CHAPTER THREE

6. Mary P. Ryan, *Womanhood in America* (New York: Franklin Watts, New Viewpoints Book, 1975).

7. Ann Oakley, *Woman's Work, The Housewife, Past and Present,* (New York: Random House Vintage Book, 1976), p. 49.

8. Cynthia Fuchs Epstein, *Woman's Place* (University California Press, 1970), p. 43.

9. De Beauvoir, *Second Sex,* pp. 404, 430.

10. Welds' study quoted in syndicated Newhouse News Service article by Susan Fogg, 1977.

11. Sidney Cornelia Callahan, *The Working Mother* (New York: Macmillan Co., 1971), pp. 31, 46.

12 Sheila D. Collins, *A Different Heaven and Earth* (Valley Forge, Pa.: Judson Press, 1974), p. 161.

13. Pierre Teilhard de Chardin, *The Divine Milieu* (New York: Harper & Bros., 1960), p. 41.

14. Quoted in Studs Terkel, *Working* (New York: Pantheon Books, 1972), pp. 467–68.

15. Ibid., p. 470.

16. Ibid., pp. 521, 524.

17. Samuel C. Florman, "Engineering and the Female Mind," *Harper's,* February 1978, p. 60.

18. Study quoted in Mary Kathleen Benet, *The Secretarial Ghetto* (New York: McGraw-Hill Book Co., 1972).

19. Phyllis Chesler and Emily Jane Goodman, *Women, Money & Power* (New York: Bantam Books, 1976), p. 3.

20. Quoted in Jean Tepperman, *Not Servants, Not Machines: Office Workers Speak Out* (Boston: Beacon Press, 1976), p. 13.

21. Benet, op. cit., p. 72.

22. Ibid., p. 159.

23. Louise Kapp Howe, *Pink Collar Workers, Inside the World of Women's Work* (New York: Avon Books, 1977, 1978), p. 234.

24. Chesler, *Women, Money & Power,* p. 192. See also, Doris B. Gold, "Women and Voluntarism," in *Woman in Sexist Society,* eds. Vivian Gornick & Barbara Moran (New York: New American Library, Signet Book, 1971), pp. 546–50.

25. Amelie Oskenberg Rorty, quoted in *Working It Out,* eds. Sara Ruddick and Pamela Daniels (New York: Pantheon Books, 1977), p. 47.

26. Erica Jong, interview.

27. Cynthia Fuchs Epstein, "Bringing Women In: Rewards, Punishments, and the Structure of Achievement," in *Women and Success, The Anatomy of Achievement,* ed. Ruth Kundsin (New York: Wm. Morrow & Co., 1974), p. 16.

28. Ibid., p. 19.

29. Robin Lakoff in *Language and Women's Place* (New York: Harper & Row, 1975), and in "Women's Styles of Speaking," unpublished material.

30. Chesler, op. cit., pp. 10–11.

31. Margaret Hennig and Anne Jardin, *The Managerial Woman* (Garden City: Doubleday Anchor Press, 1977), pp. 178–80.

32. Jean Baker Miller, *New Psychology of Women,* pp. 126, 131.

33. Rosemary Ruether, quoted in Sidney Callahan, *The Working Mother,* pp. 94–95.

34. Rosemary Ruether, "Home and Work: Women's Roles and the Transformation of Values," in *Woman: New Dimensions,* ed. Walter J. Burkhardt, S.J. (Ramsey, N.J.: Paulist Press, 1977), p. 82.

35. Denise Levertov, "Prayer for Revolutionary Love," in *The Freeing of the Dust* (New York: New Directions Books, 1975), p. 97.

THE LEGEND

1. Bettelheim, *Uses of Enchantment,* pp. 221–22.

2. Elizabeth Ashley, quoted in *Three Women Alone,* ed. Betty Lyons (New York: Award Books, 1974), pp. 143–44.

3. Eugene Hammel, "The Myth of Structural Analysis: Levi-Strauss and the Three Bears," Addison-Wesley Module in Anthropology (Menlo Park, Cal.: Cummings Publishing Co., 1972), p. 14.

4. Ibid., p. 22.

5. Bettelheim, op. cit., p. 222.

6. Dorothy Dinnerstein, *The Mermaid and the Minotaur, Sexual Arrangements and the Human Malaise* (New York: Harper & Row, 1976), pp. 9, 12, 22.

CHAPTER FOUR

7. Jean Houston, "Re-seeding America: The American Psyche as a Garden of Delights," *Journal of Humanistic Psychology,* Vol. 18, No. 1, Winter, 1978, pp. 7–8.

8. Michael Young, Peter Willmott, *The Symmetrical Family* (New York: Pantheon Books, 1973), p. 278.

9. Dorothy Dinnerstein, *The Mermaid and the Minotaur,* pp. 176, 186.

10. Ibid., pp. 77, 89.

11. Ibid., pp. 66–67.

12. Philip Slater, *Footholds* (New York: E. P. Dutton, 1977), pp. 29–30.

13. Ibid., pp. 15–16.

14. Lawrence Stone, "The Rise of the Nuclear Family in Early Modern England: The Patriarchal Stage," in *The Family in History,* ed. Charles Rosenberg (University of Pennsylvania Press, 1975), pp. 28 et passim.

15. Herbert W. Richardson, *Nun, Witch, Playmate: The Americanization of Sex* (New York: Harper & Row, 1971), p. 34.

16. Pierre Teilhard de Chardin, *The Phenomenon of Man* (New York: Harper & Row Torchbook, 1959), p. 262.

17. Paul Tillich, *Systematic Theology,* Vol. II, pp. 71–72.

18. Penelope Washbourn, *Becoming Woman: The Quest for Wholeness in Female Experience* (New York: Harper & Row, 1977), p. 30.

19. Joyce Sunila, "Women and Mr. Goodbar," *Human Behavior,* March 1978, p. 65.

20. Midge Decter, "Toward the New Chastity," *Atlantic Monthly,* October 1972, p. 55.

21. Albert Camus, *Notebooks, 1942–1951,* trans. Justin O'Brien (New York: Harcourt Brace Jovanovich, Harvest Book, 1978), pp. 36–37.

22. Margaret Adams, *Single Blessedness* (Middlesex, Eng.: Penguin Books, 1978), p. 163.

23. Ibid., p. 168.

24. Ibid., pp. 81, 82.

25. Ashley, in *Three Women Alone,* p. 144.

26. Judith Thurman, "Living Alone," *Ms.* magazine, July 1975, pp. 64–65.

27. Robert Jay Lifton, *Boundaries, Psychological Man in Revolution* (New York: Random House Vintage Book, 1967), pp. 44, 47.

28. Pierre Teilhard de Chardin, *Letters to Two Friends, 1926–1952* (Cleveland: World Publishing Co., Meridian Book, 1969), pp. 83, 88.

29. Ernest Hemingway, "In Another Country," *The Snows of Kili-*

manjaro and Other Stories (New York: Charles Scribner's Sons, 1970 [reprint]), p. 69.

30. Stanton Peele, *Love and Addiction* (New York: New American Library Signet Book, 1975), pp. 72, 124.

31. Ibid., pp. 185–86.

32. Rollo May, *The Courage to Create* (New York: Bantam Books, Inc., 1975), pp. 12–13.

33. Margaret Atwood, *Surfacing* (New York: Popular Library, 1972, 1976), p. 55.

34. Nena O'Neill, *The Marriage Premise* (New York: M. Evans & Co., 1977), p. 88.

35. David Cooper, *The Death of the Family* (New York: Pantheon Books, 1970), p. 35.

36. R. D. Laing, *The Politics of the Family and Other Essays* (New York: Random House Vintage Book, 1969).

37. Ibid., pp. 78, 87, 15, 14.

38. Christopher Lasch, *Haven in a Heartless World* (New York: Basic Books, 1977), p. 141.

39. Atwood, op. cit., pp. 221, 222, 224.

40. Philip Rieff, *The Triumph of the Therapeutic* (New York: Harper & Row, 1966), p. 243.

41. Washbourn, op. cit., p. 74.

42. Kingsley Davis, quoted in Michael Gordon. *The American Family: Past, Present and Future* (New York: Random House, 1978), p. 305.

43. Gabriel Marcel, *Creative Fidelity* (New York: Farrar, Straus and Co., 1964), p. 163.

44. Samuel Terrien, "Toward a Biblical Theology of Womanhood," in *Male and Female, Christian Approaches to Sexuality,* ed. Ruth Tiffany Barnhouse and Urban T. Holmes, III (New York: Seabury Press, 1976), p. 24.

45. Ronald Mazur, *The New Intimacy* (Boston: Beacon Press, 1973), p. 88.

46. Maria Isabel Barreno, Maria Teresa Horta, Maria Velho da Costa, *The Three Marias: New Portuguese Letters,* trans. Helen Lane (Garden City: Doubleday & Co., Inc., 1975), pp. 139, 142.

THE LEGEND

1. Bettelheim, *Uses of Enchantment,* p. 308.

2. Anaïs Nin, *Seduction of the Minotaur* (Chicago: Swallow Press, 1961; reissue 1972), p. 111.

3. Erich Neumann, *Amor and Psyche, The Psychic Development of the Feminine,* trans. Ralph Manheim (Princeton University Press, 1956; reissue 1971), pp. 78–80.

4. Ibid., p. 143.

5. Jean Cocteau, *La Belle et La Bête, Scenario et Dialogues* (New York University Press, 1970), pp. 242, 268, 354.

CHAPTER FIVE

6. Friday, *My Mother/My Self,* p. 115.

7. Bernard Meland, *The Realities of Faith* (Oxford University Press, 1962), p. 241.

8. De Chardin, *Toward the Future,* pp. 117–29.

9. Ibid., pp. 119–20.

10. L. J. Lebret, quoted in Denis Goulet, *A New Moral Order* (Maryknoll, N.Y.: Orbis Books, 1974), p. 41.

11. Tillich, *Systematic Theology,* III, p. 266.

12. Ibid., p. 271.

13. Washbourn, *Becoming Woman,* p. 97.

14. Irene Claremont de Castillejo, *Knowing Woman, A Feminine Psychology* (New York: Harper & Row, 1974), p. 94.

15. Paul W. Rahmeier, "Abortion and the Reverence for Life," in *Current Issues in Marriage and the Family,* ed. J. Gipson Wells (New York: Macmillan Co., 1975), pp. 184–92. See also Joseph F. Donceel, "Immediate Animation and Delayed Hominization," *Theological Studies,* 31:76–105 (March 1970).

16. Adrienne Rich, *Of Woman Born, Motherhood as Experience and Institution* (New York: W. W. Norton, 1976), p. 176.

17. Quoted in Ibid., pp. 179–80.

18. Washbourn, op. cit., p. 125.

19. Dante Alighieri, *The Inferno,* trans. John Ciardi (New York: New American Library Mentor Classic, 1954), p. 28.

20. M. Esther Harding, "The Value and Meaning of Depression," Paper presented to the Analytical Psychology Club of New York, 1970, p. 1.

21. Chesler, *Women and Madness,* pp. 44–45.

22. Soren Kierkegaard, *Sickness Unto Death,* trans. Walter Lowrie (Princeton University Press, 1941; reissue 1970), p. 208.

23. Harding, op. cit., p. 16.

24. Chesler, op. cit., p. 56.

25. Gregory Bateson in R. D. Laing, *The Politics of Experience* (New York: Ballantine Books, 1971), pp. 118ff.

26. Juan Luis Segundo, S.J., *A Theology for Artisans of a New Humanity,* Vol. IV (Maryknoll, N.Y.: Orbis Books, 1974), p. 33.

27. Nicolas Berdyaev, *The Meaning of the Creative Act,* trans. Donald Lowrie (London: Victor Gollancz, Ltd., 1955), p. 18.

28. Sheldon Kopp, *If You Meet Buddha on the Road, Kill Him!* (New York: Bantam Books, 1976), p. 188.

29. Rosemary Radford Ruether, "Sexism and God-talk," in *Women & Men: the Consequences of Power,* Selected Papers from the Bicentennial Conference, "Pioneers for Century III," April 1976, Cincinnati, O., ed. Dana Hiller, Robin Sheets (Office of Women's Studies, University of Cincinnati), pp. 409–10.

30. Ibid., p. 411.

31. Julia O'Faolain, Lauro Martines, eds., *Not in God's Image* (New York: Harper & Row Torchbook, 1973), p. 130.

32. John F. Haught, *Religion and Self-Acceptance* (Ramsey, N.J.: Paulist Press, 1976), pp. 156–58. See also, Nicolas Berdyaev, *Slavery and Freedom,* trans. fr. Russian by R. M. French (New York: Charles Scribner's Sons, 1944), p. 85.

33. Segundo, op. cit., Vol. III, pp. 155, 179.

34. C. G. Jung, *Memories, Dreams Reflections,* ed. Aniela Jaffee, trans. Richard and Clara Winston (New York: Pantheon Books, 1963), p. 39.

35. Eugene O'Neill, *Strange Interlude* (London: Jonathan Cape, 1928) Act II, p. 76.

36. Juliane of Norwich, *A Shewing of God's Love* (London: Sheed & Ward, 1958; reissue 1974), ed. Anna Maria Reynolds, pp. 82, 84.

37. Elaine H. Pagels, "What Became of God the Mother? Conflicting Images of God in Early Christianity," *Signs: Journal of Women in Culture and Society,* Winter, 1976, Vol. 2, No. 2, pp. 293–303.

38. Ruether, "Sexism and God-talk," p. 413.

39. J. Preston Cole, *The Problematic Self in Kierkegaard and Freud* (Yale University Press, 1971), p. 227.

40. Carol Ochs, *Behind the Sex of God* (Boston: Beacon Press, 1977), Ch. 7.

41. Carol P. Christ, "The New Feminist Theology: A Review of the Literature," *Religious Studies Review,* Vol. 3, No. 4, October 1977, p. 211.

42. Jacques Pasquier, "Experience and Conversion," *The Way,* 17:2 (April 1977), p. 115.

43. Ochs, op. cit., p. 121.

44. Berdyaev, *Slavery and Freedom,* pp. 83–84.

45. P. Ricoeur, quoted in Donald Gelpi, *Experiencing God* (Ramsey, N.J.: Paulist Press, 1978), p. 207.

46. Gregory Baum, *Man Becoming, God in Secular Experience* (New York: Seabury Press, 1970), p. 160.

47. Segundo, op. cit., Vol. III, p. 181.
48. Tillich, op. cit., III, p. 294.
49. Cole, op. cit., p. 228.
50. Cole, loc. cit.
51. Berdyaev, *The Meaning of the Creative Act,* pp. 107, 320. See also pp. 105, 332.
52. Ronald Duska, Mariellen Whelan, *A Guide to Piaget and Kohlberg* (Ramsey, N.J.: Paulist Press, 1975), and Donald Gelpi, *Experiencing God.*
53. Jim Fowler and Sam Keen, *Life Maps: Conversations on the Journey of Faith,* pp. 96–99.
54. Segundo, op. cit., Vol. IV, pp. 35–36.
55. Valerie Saiving Goldstein, "The Human Situation: A Feminine Viewpoint," *The Nature of Man in Theological and Psychological Perspective,* ed. Simon Doniger (New York: Harper & Row, 1962), p. 165.
56. G. Palmer Pardington, III, "The Holy Ghost is Dead—The Holy Spirit Lives," in *Religious Experience and Process Theology,* ed. Harry J. Cargas and Bernard Lee (Ramsey, N.J.: Paulist Press, 1976), pp. 123–24.
57. Dag Hammarskjold, *Markings,* trans. Leif Sjoberg & W. H. Auden (New York: Alfred A. Knopf, 1965), p. 106.
58. Segundo, op. cit., Vol. III, p. 39.
59. Berdyaev, *The Meaning of the Creative Act,* p. 189.
60. Ochs, op. cit., p. 68.
61. Rosemary Radford Ruether, *Mary—The Feminine Face of the Church* (Philadelphia: Westminster Press, 1977), p. 18.
62. Robert Briffault, *The Mothers,* abridged, Gordon Rattray Taylor (New York: Atheneum, 1977), p. 429.
63. Elizabeth Gould Davis, *The First Sex* (Middlesex, Eng.: Penguin Books, 1971), p. 244.
64. Wolfgang Lederer, *The Fear of Women* (New York: Harcourt Brace Jovanovich, 1968), p. 174.
65. Ruether, "Sexism and God-talk," p. 421.
66. C. G. Jung, *Psychological Reflections,* ed. Jolande Jacobi (Princeton University Press, 1953; reissue 1974), p. 99.
67. Lederer, op. cit., p. 179.

THE LEGEND

1. Julius E. Heuscher, *A Psychiatric Study of Fairy Tales* (Springfield, Ill.: Charles C. Thomas Pub., 1963), p. 91.
2. Anne Sexton, *Transformations* (New York: Houghton Mifflin, 1971), pp. 93–94.

3. Bruno Bettelheim, *Uses of Enchantment,* p. 288.
4. Ibid., p. 289.

EPILOGUE

The author acknowledges indebtedness for portions of this chapter to the following:

Eugene Bianchi and Rosemary Radford Ruether, *From Machismo to Mutuality* (Ramsey, N.J.: Paulist Press, 1976).

Glen Bucher, *Straight, White, Male* (Philadelphia: Fortress Press, 1976).

Warren Farrell, *The Liberated Man* (New York: Bantam Books, Inc., 1975).

Marc Feigen Fasteau, *The Male Machine* (New York: McGraw-Hill, 1974).

Herb Goldberg, *The Hazards of Being Male* (New York: New American Library Signet Book, 1977).

Brendan E. A. Liddell, "Before Androgyny: An Examination of the Stages Toward Neo-Masculinity," in *Women and Men: The Consequences of Power,* ed. Dana Hiller & Robin Sheets (University of Cincinnati, 1977), pp. 369–70.

INDEX